Y0-BCR-316

COLOR ATLAS
OF ORAL
MANIFESTATIONS
OF AIDS

COLOR ATLAS OF ORAL MANIFESTATIONS OF AIDS

SOL SILVERMAN, Jr., M.A., D.D.S.
Professor of Oral Medicine
University of California, San Francisco

SECOND EDITION

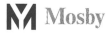 Mosby

St. Louis Baltimore Boston
Carlsbad Chicago Naples New York Philadelphia Portland
London Madrid Mexico City Singapore Sydney Tokyo Toronto Wiesbaden

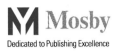
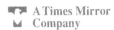

Publisher: Don Ladig
Executive Editor: Linda L. Duncan
Developmental Editor: Penny Rudolph
Project Manager: Peggy Fagen
Editorial Assistant: Kimberly Washington
Manufacturing Supervisor: Linda Ierardi
Art Director: Kay Kramer
Electronic Production Coordinator: Joan Herron

SECOND EDITION

Copyright © 1996 by Mosby–Year Book, Inc.

Previous edition copyrighted 1989

Printed in the United States of America

Typesetting by Mosby Electronic Production
Printing and binding by Grafos, Barcelona

Mosby–Year Book, Inc.
11830 Westline Industrial Drive
St. Louis, MO 63146

International Standard Book Number 0-8151-7897-2

95 96 97 98 99 / 9 8 7 6 5 4 3 2 1

PREFACE

Although it is now well into the second decade of the AIDS pandemic, there is yet no end in sight. For families and for nations, the disaster continues. Human immunodeficiency virus infections and reported cases of AIDS are at all-time highs worldwide, and without an effective vaccine or viral-killing drug, the reservoir and risk for transmission increase. Mutations leading to the many strains of virus further complicate control.

Education in an attempt to alter high-risk behavior is still the principal means of controlling the spread of infections caused by the AIDS virus. Success has been far from optimal as new infections throughout the world continue. Communities and countries have been devastated as the fastest increasing spread has shifted from the homosexual to the heterosexual population. Unidentified HIV partners, prostitution, and the use of illegal/recreational drugs have been main factors.

This atlas has been updated to illustrate the numerous opportunistic infections, HIV-associated malignancies, and immunologic conditions that affect the mouth and involve oral health care professionals. Illustrations have been increased to facilitate recognition of the variety of forms of oral manifestations, and the text has been expanded and updated for diagnostic and treatment approaches. Important information regarding epidemiology, demographics, HIV biology, transmission, and pathogenesis has been summarized to give the reader an understandable background to better comprehend the clinical lesions and progression. Current key references have been added for documentation and further reading if desired.

Sol Silverman, Jr.

CONTENTS

1   THE NATURE OF HIV INFECTION

EPIDEMIOLOGY

Now well into the second decade, acquired immunodeficiency syndrome (AIDS) continues to spread throughout the world without any end in sight. By 1995, AIDS, the terminal phase of human immunodeficiency virus (HIV) infection as defined by 27 AIDS-defining diseases/conditions, has been estimated by the World Health Organization (WHO) to have afflicted over 4 million persons in more than 179 nations. Some examples of AIDS-defining disorders include CD4 counts less than 200, candidal esophagitis, Kaposi's sarcoma, *Pneumocystis carinii* pneumonia, and the progressive wasting syndrome. Furthermore, the WHO estimates that about 17 million individuals throughout the world are HIV-infected. Most cases have been reported in sub-Sahara Africa, but the fastest increase seems to be in southeast Asia.

The United States has the largest number of reported AIDS cases compared to all other countries. By mid 1995, over 450,000 cases had been recorded by the Centers for Disease Control and Prevention (CDC), the national repository for information on infectious diseases in the United States. In 1995, more than 1300 new cases of AIDS were being reported each week. Comparing this number with a similar period in 1994, there seemed to be a leveling-off of newly reported cases. The CDC has estimated that between 1 and 1.5 million Americans are probably HIV-positive. Therefore the number of HIV-infected persons forms a substantial pool for viral passage and for those who will eventually develop AIDS. Approximately 60% of those with AIDS have died, with the two most common causes being the progessive wasting syndrome and *Pneumocystis carinii* pneumonia.

AIDS is the fastest increasing cause of mortality in the United States, ranking as the sixth leading disease-cause of death. At present, AIDS is the leading cause of death in US men between the ages of 25 and 44 and the second leading disease-cause of death in US women of the same age group.

Demographics

Throughout the world, including the United States, HIV is spreading most rapidly in the heterosexual population. Thus AIDS is no longer a predominantly homosexual disease. Over half of the newly reported AIDS cases to the CDC are in heterosexuals, primarily associated with the use of illegal drugs, contaminated needles, prostitution, and unprotected sex. At present, 18% of these cases are in women. However, the number of women is increasing each year, and by the begining of the year 2000 the percentage of HIV-positive women in the United States may well approximate 40% to 50%.

As testing and processing US blood supplies improve, infections acquired through blood banks are almost nonexistent. Thus the number of newly infected hemophiliacs has decreased substantially. While infected blood also poses a small risk for infants, pediatric AIDS is mainly passed from infected mothers either in utero or during birth. Although there seems to be an underreporting problem, pediatric AIDS (up to age 13) still accounts for about 1% of the reported cases.

The mean age of newly reported AIDS cases is the third decade of life. Obviously, infection takes place much earlier. From some cohort studies, the median time from HIV infection to signs and symptoms of AIDS approximated 10 to 11 years. There is no ethnic barrier. However, there is a disproportionately large number of infected Afro-Americans and Latinos compared to their proportion of the general US population. These two ethnic groups account for over 50% of heterosexual AIDS patients while comprising only 21% of the total population.

PATHOGENESIS, TRANSMISSION, AND PROGRESSION

HIV infection is essentially 100% fatal. The uniqueness of this viral lethality is based on the fact that HIV can directly attack cells of the immune system, more specifically lymphocytes and macrophages. This initiates an eventual irreversible immune suppression, leading to AIDS-defining opportunistic infections and malignancies.

While HIV can attack any tissue in the body, it preferentially affects immune system cells because of the large number of surface receptors (CD4), which permit attachment with HIV surface glycoprotein (gp 120), enhancing host cell invasion and infection. The attack on T-lymphocytes is particularly critical, since these are the cells that modulate the immune system by cytokine production. Once cell invasion takes place, HIV polymerase gene (pol) produces the enzyme "reverse transcriptase" that allows the incorporation of HIV RNA into host nucleus genome DNA. This creates a permanent pattern and reservoir for perpetuating RNA viral copies.

The rate of this reassembly is influenced by poorly understood co-factors and proteases. While progression to the terminal phase (AIDS) may be rapid, in many infected individuals the immunosuppression is a slow process, taking many years. But as the immunosuppression continues, more host lymphocytes are killed or become physiologically hypofunctional from the increased viral load, and the host becomes more virulent to partners as well as susceptible to increasing numbers of opportunistic infections, immunologic diseases, and malignancies. While cigarette smoking seems to diminish host immune response initially, it does not appear to influence the final outcome. Neutralizing antibodies probably play an important role in the infection process.

It should be remembered that at all stages of HIV infection, even during long asymptomatic incubation periods, HIV is being produced and shed by HIV-infected patients, and those individuals are potentially infectious to partners.

SURVIVAL AND TREATMENT STRATEGIES

While many HIV-infected individuals live for many years, even more than a decade, there is little evidence to support eventual survival. HIV is a lethal infection. Staging is most commonly assessed by the number of circulating CD4 lymphocytes and AIDS-defining diseases.

Treatment strategies are based on prevention of infection and use of drugs or vaccines that will inhibit the function of key genes or proteins that contribute to viral infectivity and replication. Examples include vaccines, condoms, or viricides (vaginal foams) that will inhibit or prevent infection; antibodies against cell receptors or genes; and protease inhibitors to prevent reassembly from nuclear DNA.

HIV characteristically rapidly mutates. Because of this, there are many HIV strains, which accounts for the extreme variability in signs, symptoms, and survival. These mutations complicate viral identification and hinder progress toward developing effective vaccines and drugs. With no effective cure or preventative presently in sight, educational approaches to alter behavior patterns are essential and critical to controlling the spread of HIV.

SUGGESTED READINGS

Epidemiology and Demographics

Centers for Disease Control and Prevention: Update: AIDS Among Women—United States, 1994. MMWR 1995; 44:81-84.

Centers for Disease Control and Prevention: US HIV and AIDS Cases Reported through December 1994. HIV/AIDS Surveillance Report 1995; 6 (No 2): 5-26.

Pathogenesis, Transmission, and Progression

Coodley GO, Loveless MO, Merrill TM: The HIV Wasting Syndrome: A Review. J Acquir Immun Defic Syndr 1994; 7:681- 694.

Detels R, Liu Z, Hennessey K, et al: Resistance to HIV-1 Infection. J Acquir Immun Defic Syndr 1994; 7:1263-1269.

Diaz T, Chu SY, Conti L, et al: Risk Behaviors of Persons with Heterosexually Acquired HIV Infection in the United States: Results of a Multistate Surveillance Project. J Acquir Immun Defic Syndr 1994; 7:958-963.

Levy JA: Pathogenesis of Human Immunodeficiency Virus Infection. Microbiol Rev 1993; 57:183-289.

Panteleo G, Graziosi C, Fauci AS: The Immunopathogenesis of Human Immunodeficiency Virus Infection. N Engl J Med 1994; 328:327-335.

Park LP, Margolick JB, Giorgi JV, et al: Influence of HIV-1 Infection and Cigarette Smoking on Leukocyte Profiles in Homosexual Men. J Acquir Immun Defic Syndr 1992; 5:1124-1130.

Phair J, Jacobson L, Detels R, et al: Acquired Immune Deficiency Syndrome Occurring Within 5 Years of Infection with Human Immunodeficiency Virus Type-1: The Multicenter AIDS Cohort Study. J Acquir Immun Defic Syndr 1994; 5:490- 496.

Saag MS, Hammer SM, Lange JMA: Pathogenicity and Diversity of HIV and Implications for Clinical Management: A Review. J Acquir Immun Defic Syndr 1994; 7(Suppl. 2):S2-S11.

de Vincenzi I: A Longitudinal Study of Human Immunodeficiency Virus Transmission by Heterosexual Partners. N Engl J Med 1994; 331:341-346.

Wong-Staal F: AIDS Research: A Five-Year Perspective. J NIH Res 1994;6:71-67.

Survival and Treatment Strategies

Letvin NL: Vaccines Against Human Immunodeficiency Virus—Progress and Prospects. N Engl J Med 1993; 329:1400-1405.

Munoz A, Kirby AJ, He YD, et al: Long-Term Survivors with HIV-1 Infection: Incubation Period and Longitudinal Patterns of CD4+ Lymphocytes. J Acquir Immun Defic Syndr 1995; 8:496-505.

2 ORAL MANIFESTATIONS OF HIV INFECTION

ROLE OF CLINICIANS AND DENTAL PROFESSIONALS

Knowingly or unknowingly, HIV-infected patients are being treated in dental and other professional offices. Many times patients are not aware of their HIV status. Therefore, knowledge of HIV infection has become a critically important requirement for professionals responsible for oral health care delivery. History taking, examination, differential diagnosis, and referral have taken on new dimensions. The need for combined education and understanding of HIV infection is summarized by the following:

1. HIV-infected patients actively seek dental care.

2. Many patients are either unaware of their HIV status or may elect not to divulge this information.

3. Often oral lesions associated with HIV infection may be a chief complaint, requiring expertise in oral health care for diagnosis and treatment.

4. Not infrequently, an oral infection or neoplasm can be the first sign and/or symptom of HIV infection.

5. An increase in frequency or severity of many oral lesions in the HIV-positive patient can reflect a declining immune competency, ineffectiveness of treatment, and progression of the terminal phase.

6. Treatment of HIV patients has raised the real and emotional concerns of health care workers regarding their own safety and transmission risks.

7. Ethical and legal guidelines mandate against discrimination of providing services for known or suspected HIV-positive individuals.

8. In addition to HIV infection, there are many other transmissible infectious diseases that may pose a risk, such as tuberculosis, hepatitis, and herpes.

TRANSMISSION RISKS

Risks of transmission include clinician to patient, patient to clinician, patient to patient, and casual contact. There is little evidence to support transmission by casual contact; passage stems from sex and/or HIV-contaminated blood.

At present, there is only one documented case of doctor to patient(s) transmission. This is the case of the southern Florida dentist, Dr. Acer. Dr. Acer's HIV appears to be and probably was the virus that infected six of his patients over a 3-year period. Why these six patients became infected out of more than 1150 treated during the same time period remains an enigma. These six patients had no other known risk factors, and their viral DNA sequencing was similar to Dr. Acer's virus. How Dr. Acer's HIV was transmitted is completely unknown and probably forever will remain a mystery.

Studies of patients of more than 57 HIV-positive doctors showed no HIV transmission. Proof of passage required no high-risk patient behavior and similar DNA viral sequencing.

There are very few cases of occupational HIV infection. Over 130 such cases have been investigated by the CDC, and 42 have been proved. These instances have all been associated with needle-stick injuries or mucosal splashes. None of these cases has involved dental personnel. In the unproven health care worker seroconversions, six were dental workers, and very few involved injuries. The conclusion to be drawn is that occupational transmission is possible but not probable. At this time, there is no effective prophylaxis after exposure to known or suspected HIV-contaminated blood.

Although seroconversion has occurred when direct contact of body secretions other than through sex has taken place between HIV-positive and HIV-negative individuals, documented cases have been extremely rare (less than a dozen in the United States). Once again, this indicates a possibility with a very low probability. Patient-to-patient transmission by seronegative health care workers is extremely rare, with only one probable situation being reported. This involved an HIV-negative surgeon whose office was apparently responsible for infecting four patients who underwent invasive procedures on the same day the surgeon removed a skin cyst from an HIV-infected patient. Ineffective sterilization is suspected.

These infrequent and rare instances of seroconversion indicate the low virulence relative to infectivity of HIV. Therefore, with the use of universal precautions using barrier techniques and following proper sterilization/disinfection guidelines, clinicians, office workers, and patients should feel safe in professional offices, even during invasive procedures.

SALIVA

As already indicated, HIV transmission involves direct parenteral contact with HIV-infected body secretions, most commonly blood, semen, and vaginal fluid. Epidemiologic and family studies have failed to provide any conclusive evidence that saliva serves as a vehicle for transmission. Additionally, virus or virus particles are rarely found in the saliva of HIV-infected persons. One report indicated less than 1% of HIV-positive patients showed virus in saliva specimens. One explanation might be based on the finding of a mucin-rich (glycoprotein) fraction of saliva that has properties inhibiting HIV replication in vitro, thus modulating the infectivity of HIV. This mechanism may be due to a physical-chemical binding between the glycoprotein and the virus.

OTHER TRANSMISSIBLE DISEASES

HIV infection usually reflects a lifestyle of high-risk behavior as well as immune incompetence. Therefore, other sexually transmitted diseases occur in higher than expected frequency in this group as compared to the general population. Of greatest concern are hepatitis and herpes viruses. These are covered in Chapter 4. More recently tuberculosis has become of epidemic significance because of a rise in incidence and the emergence of drug-resistant strains. Tuberculosis is covered in Chapter 5.

DIFFERENTIAL DIAGNOSIS AND PATIENT APPROACH

As one would expect, when the immune system is compromised, an increase in opportunistic infections (fungal, viral, bacterial), malignancies, and immunologic diseases/conditions will occur. Previously known diseases may occur more frequently and with greater severity, and new oral disease problems will emerge. These manifestations can be the first sign and/or symptom of HIV infection or an indication of progressive immunosuppression. In any event, they should signal the need for HIV status evaluation. Careful examinations and history information coupled with a realistic differential diagnosis are essential. Training, experience, and judgment will determine the ordering or performing of tests/procedures and/or acceptable explanations to patients for referrals. Since the oral cavity is so commonly affected in the immunocompromised patient, knowledge of HIV infection, pathogenesis of immunodeficiency, diagnosis, significance, and management is essential for optimal care.

With the increasing number of HIV-infected women of childbearing age, there is a corresponding increase in HIV-positive newborns (about 30%). This is due to vertical transmission in utero. In HIV-infected children, the most common oral lesions are thrush, herpes, and parotid enlargement.

The following cases indicate some variable complaints and findings that raised initial suspicions of HIV infection.

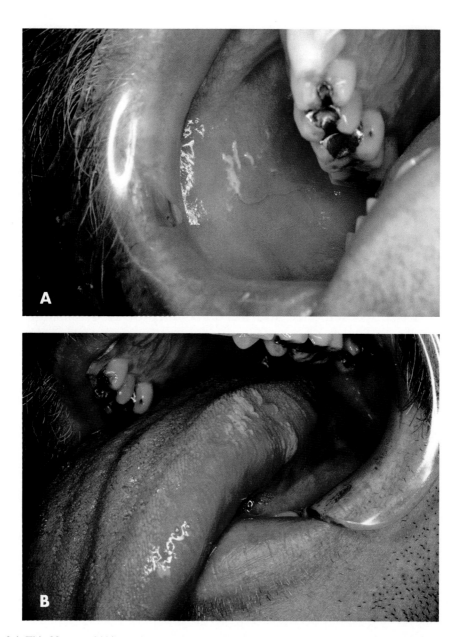

Figure 2.1 This 28-year-old bisexual man reported to the clinic for routine dental care. He acknowledged a history of gonorrhea and hepatitis B. Clinical examination revealed (1) asymptomatic surface white lesions on the buccal mucosa (**A**), which were confirmed as candidal colonies, and (2) white lesions on the lateral border of the tongue (**B**), which were confirmed as "hairy leukoplakia." Serologic testing indicated that the patient was HIV-infected.

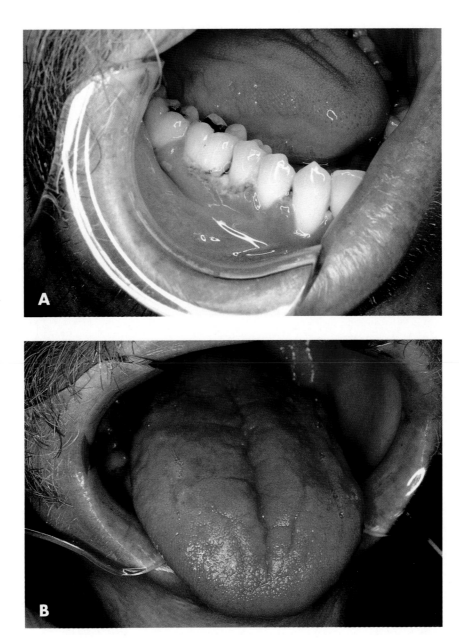

Figure 2.2 A, This 30-year-old homosexual male patient reported to our clinic because of a painful and unexplainable acute necrotizing ulcerative gingivitis. He had a history of presently controlled venereal disease and hepatitis (forms unknown). He occasionally smoked marijuana. **B,** Oral examination also revealed glossitis that was only mildly irritable. This was confirmed as caused by candidiasis. Three months later he developed a cough, and *Pneumocystis carinii* pneumonia was diagnosed. He died of AIDS 1 year later.

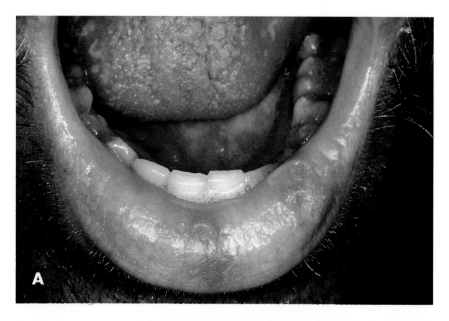

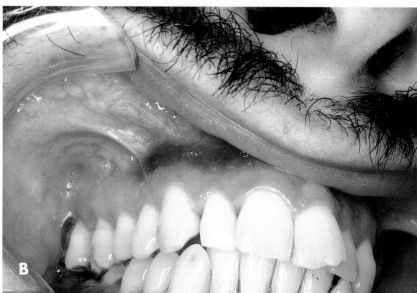

Figure 2.3 A, This 31-year-old homosexual patient sought consultation because of an increase in frequency and severity of recurrent herpes ("cold sores") associated with his lower lip. Previous to these recent bouts, he would experience two or three single-sore attacks each year. This prompted HIV testing, which resulted in a positive result. **B,** Upon examination, an asymptomatic purple-appearing lesion of the maxillary gingiva was found. A biopsy showed this to be Kaposi's sarcoma, indicating that the patient already had an AIDS-defining disease.

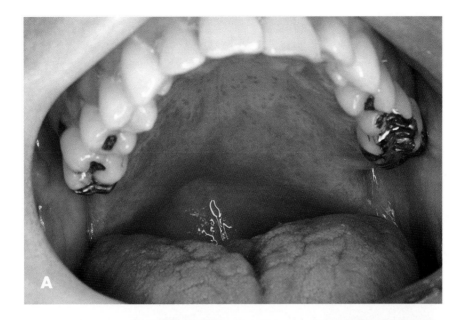

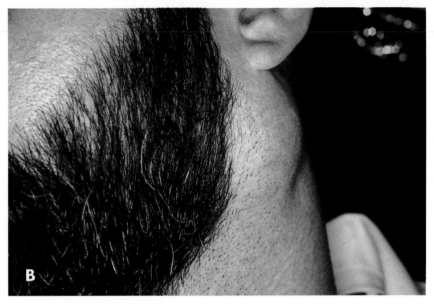

Figure 2.4 A 31-year-old bisexual male sought consultation because of palatal "irritation." His medical history was negative except for a past bout with venereal disease, recent fatigability, and slight weight loss. Clinical examination revealed the erythematous form of candidiasis on his palate (**A**) and a "lump" in the neck (**B**), which was shown to be idiopathic benign lymphadenopathy (manifestation of the "gay lymph node syndrome"). This prompted suspicion of immunosuppression, confirmed by positive HIV seroantibodies.

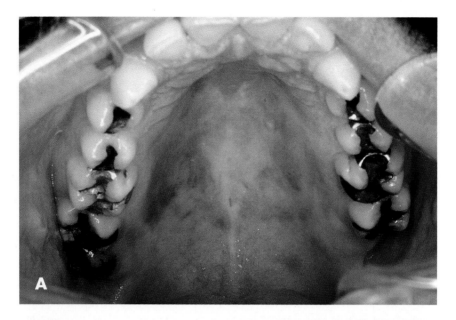

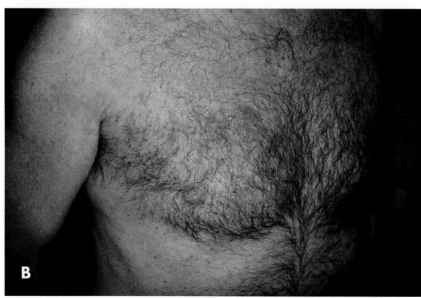

Figure 2.5 This 40-year-old homosexual male sought consultation because of a palatal discomfort. He had no other complaints except for "forgetfulness" and "hand tremors." Medical history was positive for venereal disease and occasional diarrhea caused by parasitic infections. **A,** Clinical examination revealed palatal discolorations that would not blanch upon pressure. A palatal biopsy proved the lesions to the Kaposi's sarcoma, and serology demonstrated HIV antibodies. During the next 6 months before his death, he developed zoster **(B),** erythema multiforme, progressive weakness, weight loss, and obvious leukoencephalopathy (caused by central nervous system HIV infection).

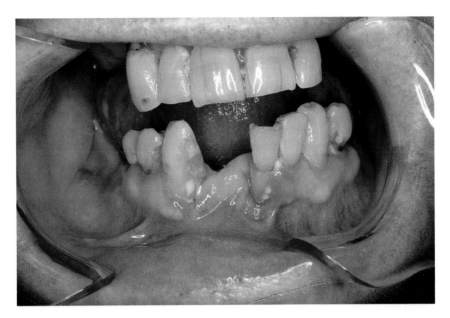

Figure 2.6 This 68-year-old man was referred because of progressive peridontal disease, oral pain, anorexia, dysgeusia, and loss of weight of 4 months' duration. Except for past angina and hypertension, the patient's medical history was negative. Because of coronary artery occlusions, bypass surgery with multiple transfusions was performed 4 years previously. He also had a mild mucosal candidiasis and HIV testing was positive. Since there was no other high-risk activity revealed, it was presumed that HIV infection was derived from the blood transfusion.

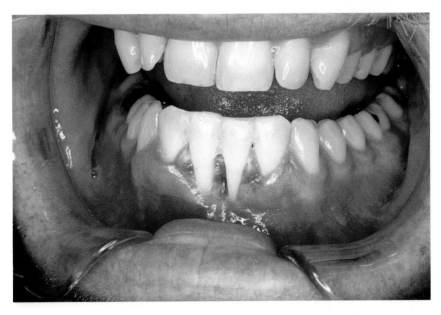

Figure 2.7 This 36-year-old bisexual man was referred because of progressive gingival recession of the lower central incisors, which was associated with pain and a granulomatous connective tissue proliferation in response to curettage. Because of suspected immunodeficiency, the patient agreed to an HIV serologic test, which resulted in a positive ELISA and Western blot, indicating HIV infection.

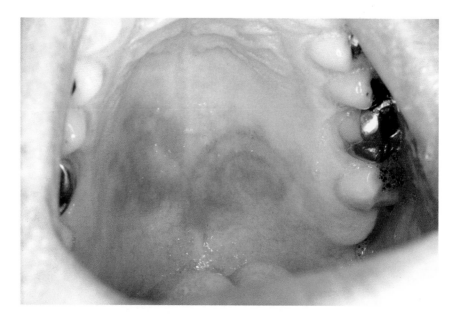

Figure 2.8 This HIV-positive patient presented with a painful palatal lesion of several days' duration. The differential diagnosis included candidiasis, a hypersensitivity reaction, or possible local irritation. The final diagnosis was inflammatory response resulting from oral sex, based on history and disappearance in 3 days without any specific treatment. A candidal smear was negative, and the patient had not used any new medications or foods.

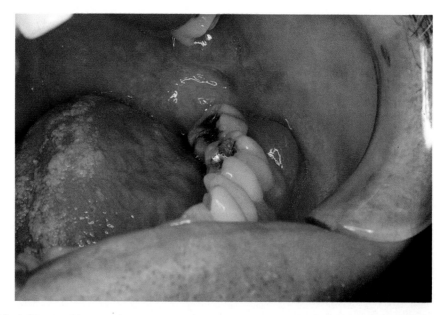

Figure 2.9 A 40-year-old gay patient was referred for assessment of a painful mandibular swelling present for 3 weeks that was unresponsive to antibiotics. Radiographs did not reveal either tooth or periodontal etiology. A biopsy showed this rubbery firm mass to be a non-Hodgkin's lymphoma (NHL). Because of the frequent association between NHL and HIV, serology was obtained and was positive for HIV infection.

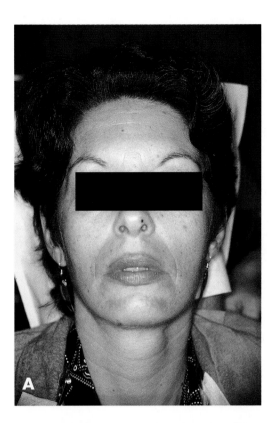

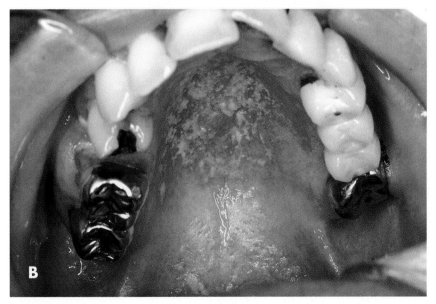

Figure 2.10 A, A 35-year-old woman, who was HIV stable for 5 years (no evidence of a declining CD4 lympho-cytes or opportunistic infections), was seen for a chief complaint of palatal discomfort. **B,** Culture diagnosis con-firmed a combination of pseudomembranous and erythematous candidiasis. A reassessment of her CD4 count showed a marked depression to less than 200 cells/μl, indicating progression to AIDS. She died the next year from pneumocystic pneumonia.

SUGGESTED READINGS

Role of Clinicians and Dental Professionals

Ficarra G, Shillitoe EJ: HIV-Related Infections of the Oral Cavity. Crit Rev Oral Biol Med 1992; 3:207-231.

Gerbert B, Bleecker T, Saub E: Risk Perception and Risk Communications: Benefits of Dentist-Patient Discussions. J Am Dent Assoc 1995; 126: 333-339.

Glick M, Muzyka C, Lurie D, Salkin LM: Oral Manifestations Associated with HIV-Related Disease as Markers for Immune Suppression and AIDS. Oral Surg Oral Med Oral Pathol 1994; 77:344-349.

Leggott PJ: Oral Manifestations of HIV Infection in Children. Oral Surg Oral Med Oral Pathol 1992; 73:187-192.

Perry SW, Moffatt M Jr, Card CAL, et al: Self-Disclosure of HIV Infection to Dentists and Physicians. J Am Dent Assoc 1993; 124:51-54.

Sadowsky D, Kunzel C: Measuring Dentists' Willingness to Treat HIV-Positive Patients. J Am Dent Assoc 1994; 125:705-710.

Transmission Risks

Beekmann SE, Henderson DK: Managing Occupational Risks in the Dental Office: HIV and the Dental Professional. J Am Dent Assoc 1994; 125:847-852.

Ciesielski CA, Marianos DW, Schochetman G, et al: The 1990 Florida Dental Investigation. Ann Intern Med 1994; 121:886- 888.

Gerberding JL: Management of Occupational Exposures to Blood-Borne Viruses. N Engl J Med 1995; 332: 444-451.

Gruninger SE, Siew C, Chang S-B, et al: Human Immunodeficiency Virus Type 1 Infection Among Dentists. J Am Dent Assoc 1992; 123:57-64.

Myers G: Molecular Investigation of HIV Transmission. Ann Intern Med 1994; 121:889:890.

Robert LM, Bell DM: HIV Transmission in the Health-Care Setting: Risks to Health-Care Workers and Patients. Infect Dis Clin N Am 1994; 8:319-328.

Siew C, Chang S-B, Bruninger SE, et al: Self-Reported Percutaneous Injuries in Dentists: Implications for HBV, HIV Transmission Risk. J Am Dent Assoc 1992; 123:37-44.

Saliva

Barr CE, Miller LK, Lopez MR, et al: Recovery of Infectious HIV-1 from Whole Saliva. J Am Dent Assoc 1992; 123:37-48.

Bergey EJ, Cho M-I, Blumberg BM, et al: Interaction of HIV-1 and Human Salivary Mucins. J Acquir Immun Defic Syndr 1994; 7:995-1002.

Coppenhaver DH, Sriyuktasuth-Woo P, Barr CE, et al: Correlation of Nonspecific Antiviral Activity with the Ability to Isolate Infectious HIV-1 from Saliva. N Engl J Med 1994; 330:1314-1315.

Moore BE, Flaitz CM, Coppenhaver DH, et al: HIV Recovery from Saliva Before and After Dental Treatment: Inhibitors May Have Critical Role in Viral Inactivation. J Am Dent Assoc 1993;124:67-74.

Yeh C-K, Handelman B, Fox PC, Baum BJ: Further Studies of Salivary Inhibition of HIV-1 Infectivity. J Acquir Immun Defic Syndr 1992; 5:898-903.

Differential Diagnosis and Patient Approach

Glick M: Guidelines for the Evaluation and Management of Early HIV Infection. J Am Coll Dent 1994; 61:5-11.

Lamster IB, Begg MD, Mitchell-Lewis D, et al: Oral Manifestations of HIV Infection in Homosexual Men and Intravenous Drug Users: Study Design and Relationship of Epidemiologic, Clinical, and Immunologic Parameters to Oral Lesions. Oral Surg Oral Med Oral Pathol 1994; 78:163-174.

3 FUNGAL INFECTIONS

CANDIDIASIS (CANDIDOSIS)

Candidal fungi are commonly found as part of the oral microbial flora. Therefore, it is not surprising that candidal overgrowth is the most common infection in HIV-positive individuals. The significance of oral candidiasis is great:

1. Many times candidal infection can be the first sign or symptom of HIV infection.

2. Often patients will present with oral candidiasis as their chief complaint, requiring recognition and treatment.

3. Candidiasis may cause discomfort or pain, halitosis, and altered taste (dysgeusia).

4. It may signal the decline of a heretofore fairly stable immune function and may even indicate an acceleration of the terminal phase of infection and shortened longevity.

5. In a known HIV patient, esophageal candidiasis is an AIDS-defining disease.

6. Candidal organisms are transmissible to immunodeficient partners.

Clinical Features

While recognition and treatment are important, they may be somewhat difficult. Signs and symptoms often do not coincide and the appearance can be variable. Commonly, the fungal infection will appear as surface white changes that frequently can be scraped off the mucosa. This is referred to as the pseudomembranous form or thrush. However, but rarely, a candidal white form cannot be removed and may be mistaken for a form of leukoplakia. This is referred to as the hyperplastic form. Candidiasis can also present as irregular, often ill-defined erythematous patches. Frequently, both white and red components are found. In many cases, with or without oral manifestations, angular cheilitis (red or white fissured lesions) will be present.

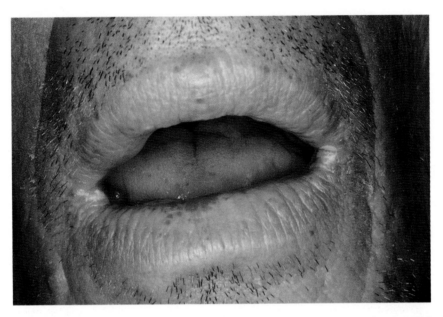

Figure 3.1 Angular cheilitis in a 60-year-old homosexual male. This was the first sign of oral candidiasis and HIV infection, the latter proved by positive serology.

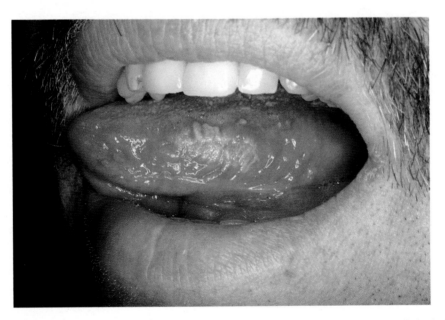

Figure 3.2 Angular cheilitis and hyperplastic candidiasis of the tongue, in this case mimicking "hairy leukoplakia." This 38-year-old bisexual business executive was not aware that he was HIV-positive and it was this finding that prompted HIV testing.

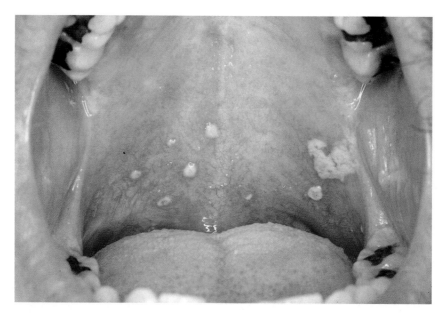

Figure 3.3 Pseudomembranous form of candidiasis in a 34-year-old AIDS patient.

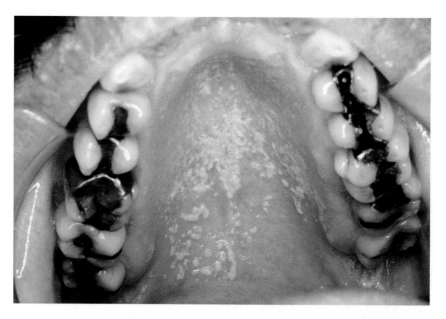

Figure 3.4 Florid candidiasis in an AIDS patient. Complaints include pain, bad breath, and altered taste.

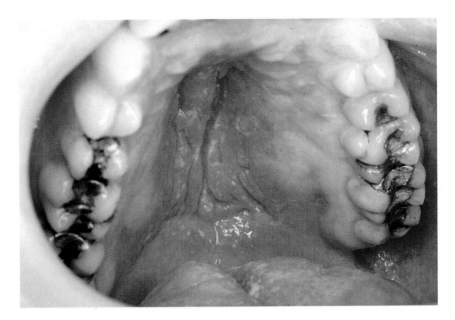

Figure 3.5 Erythematous form of candidiasis with minimal white-appearing surface colonies associated with AIDS. Palatal pain prompted the office visit.

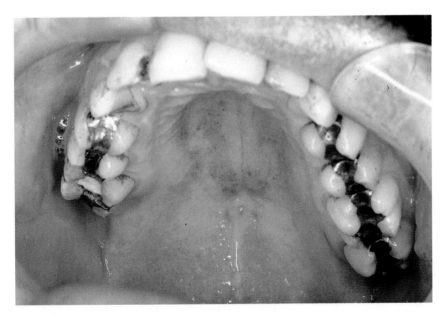

Figure 3.6 The erythematous form of candidal infection resembling telangiectatic lesions of the palate in an AIDS patient.

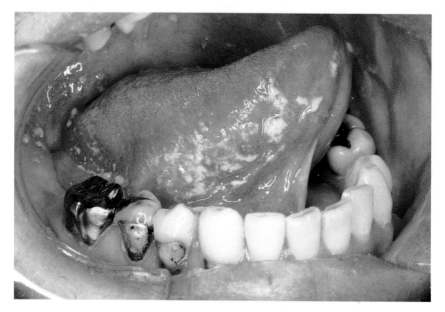

Figure 3.7 Pseudomembranous candidiasis in a 26-year-old HIV patient.

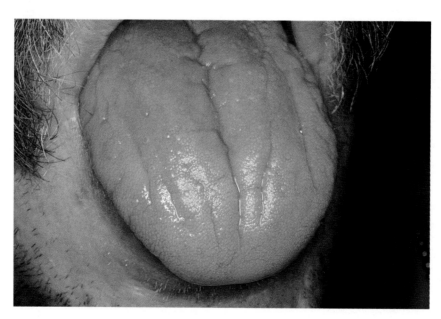

Figure 3.8 This AIDS patient sought consultation because of a severe burning sensation of the tongue associated with the atrophic form of candidiasis. Antifungal treatment reversed the signs and symptoms.

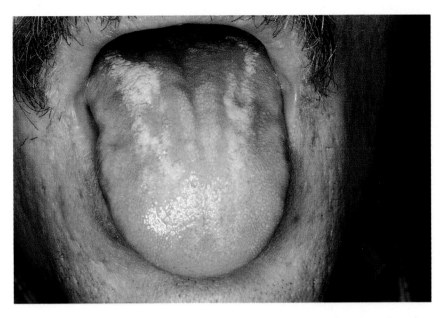

Figure 3.9 Lingual candidiasis causing an abnormal pattern of filiform papillae and surface fungal colonies. Smears were positive for *Candida*. Signs returned to normal following antifungal medication, and further scrapings tested negative.

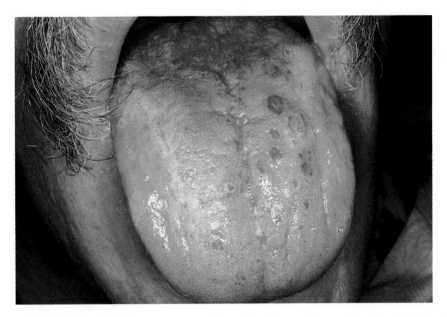

Figure 3.10 Candidal tongue lesions that at first were thought to be possible manifestations of a blood dyscrasia or a peculiar form of glossitis migrans.

Diagnosis

Sometimes the lesions are so characteristic that antifungal treatment can be started immediately to give the patient relief and retrospectively confirm the diagnosis, depending on the response. When there is clinical uncertainty, a potassium hydroxide–processed smear enables visualization of spores, hyphae, or mycelia. Cultures of lesions or saliva can be processed on dextrose-agar plates in order to determine if fungal colonies are formed. If growth occurs, the fungi can be speciated (metabolic reactions to carbohydrates) as well as quantitated by colony-forming units. If a biopsy is performed for other reasons, the presence of candidal hyphae or spores can be confirmed utilizing periodic acid Schiff stain (PAS). When present, candidal epithelial invasion between and within squamous cells is superficial. Systemic candidemia is rare.

Speciation usually is not indicated, since over 90% of oral candidiasis involves *C. albicans*. The rare occurrence of other strains is usually of little importance in treatment responses. Infection by more than one fungal strain is very rare. Presence of candidal organisms in the oral flora alone does not infer infection. Pathogenicity depends on mucosal immunity and adhesion factors, which in turn form the basis for signs and symptoms.

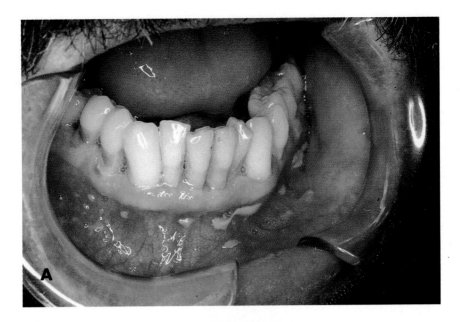

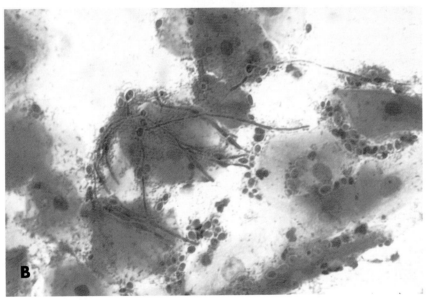

Figure 3.11 A, Gingival and mucosal candidiasis in a 30-year-old HIV patient who also had precocious periodontal disease. The mucosal lesions resembled somewhat those of a hypersensitivity reaction (erythema multiforme). **B,** A gingivolabial smear from the patient in **A** revealed hyphae, mycelia, and spores consistent with a fungal infection (Gram stain). Note the background of squamous cells. The lesions cleared with antifungal therapy.

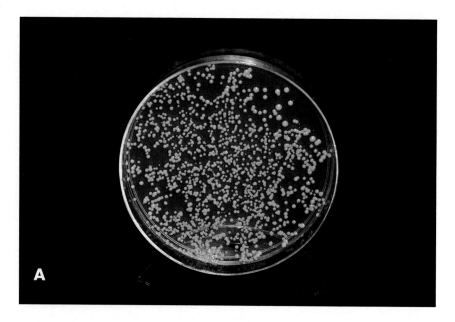

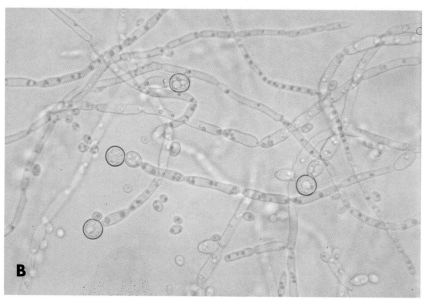

Figure 3.12 A, A culture positive for *Candida albicans.* Note the white fungal colonies grown on Sabouraud's dextrose agar. **B,** Smear of a white colony seen in **A** and observed microscopically. Note classical candidal pseudomycelia and chlamydospores.

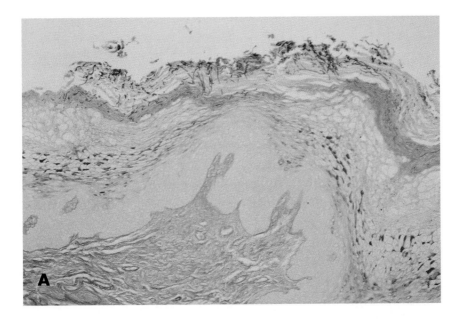

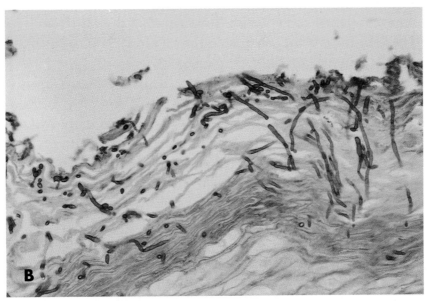

Figure 3.13 **A,** Mucosal biopsy from a patient with oral candidiasis. **B,** Higher power demonstrating various candidal forms growing in the superficial cell layers of the stratified squamous epithelium. Stained by the periodic acid Schiff method.

Treatment

Antifungal therapy can include systemic and/or topical agents. If there is patient compliance, both forms are effective, even when CD4 counts are quite low. Problems arise, however, since the mouth is usually never completely sterilized for *Candida* and recurrences are common. Additionally, even when the oral flora can be cleared of *Candida,* reinfection from the gastrointestinal tract or from partners frequently occurs.

Topical approaches primarily involve the use of nystatin or clotrimazole. Nystatin vaginal troches (100,000 U) can be effective if slowly dissolved in the mouth then swallowed three to five times daily. The suspension (500,000 U/ teaspoonful) is often not effective because of limited contact time with the mucosa. Gut absorption is very poor. Clotrimazole vaginal tablets (100 mg) are very effective, requiring only one or two to be dissolved orally then swallowed daily. The "oral" form of clotrimazole is Mycelex. While the taste is acceptable, effectiveness is limited because of the low 10 mg concentration. Also, tablets contain sugar to improve patient acceptance. Five per day dissolved orally is recommended. These forms are not acceptable for candidal esophagitis. Allergies and toxicity are uncommon.

Systemic strategies are often more successful for initial attacks or flares because of higher concentrations and better patient compliance. Ketoconazole (Nizoral) is very effective. Usually 200 or 400 mg once daily will control oral signs and symptoms. It must be taken with food or beverage to lower gastric pH (increase acidity), which is essential for optimal absorption. Since ketoconazole is metabolized in the liver, attention must be paid if there is a history of hepatitis. Allergies are uncommon. Fungal "resistance" often can be overcome by doubling the dose.

Fluconazole (Diflucan) is a very effective antifungal and is the drug of choice for candidal esophagitis. Usually 100 mg daily will control an attack. While allergies and toxicity are rare, resistant strains are often reported. Advantages involve better absorption, metabolism by the kidney, and prolonged salivary levels.

With extended usage of either systemic agent, there is a chance for fungal switching mechanisms and drug resistance. Therefore, a clinical dilemma exists on the duration of usage. Dosages for 1 to 2 weeks are common. Based on frequent recurrences, some patients chronically remain on antifungal medications. In any event, combinations of topical and systemic antifungals are used frequently, depending on patient responses and HIV status.

Amphotericin B is a very effective antifungal, but in the United States it only can be used intravenously. It is nephrotoxic, which also limits usage. Usefulness as a mouth rinse has not been documented. Antiseptic mouth rinses can be helpful as adjuncts. These include 0.12% chlorhexidine (Peridex and PerioGard) and Listerine (mixture of essential oils: thymol, eucalyptol, methyl salicylate, menthol). Since these rinses contain alcohol, "burning" sensations may limit their usage. Some usefulness may be obtained from a mixture of 3% hydrogen peroxide in equal parts warm saline.

HIV patients often are taking bacterial antibiotics for a variety of infections. Fungal growth is nurtured by these antibiotics, which reduce bacterial flora, thereby reducing competition for substrate. Also, many HIV patients suffer from xerostomia and hypofunctioning salivary glands. This diminished salivary production (and probable loss of salivary enzymes needed to control fungal reproduction) encourages candidal overgrowth. Therefore, attention must be paid to keeping the mouth moist. Frequent water rinses and sucking or chewing sugarless candy/gum are helpful. Sialogogues (salivary stimulants) are often even more effective. Pilocarpine tablets (5 mg three to four times daily) or bethanechol tablets (25 to 50 mg three times daily) can be extremely helpful in controlling recurrences.

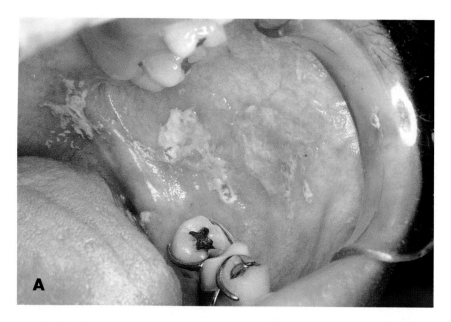

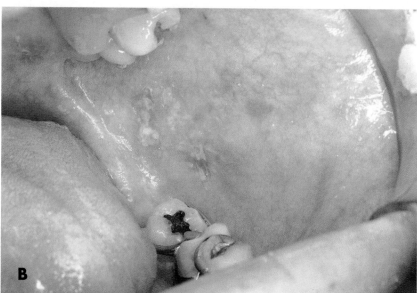

Figure 3.14 A, A mixture of pseudomembranous and hyperplastic candidiasis in a 42-year-old bisexual man. This was the initial complaint that led to the diagnosis of HIV infection. **B,** Topical antifungal medication led to partial clearing in 1 week. However, the patient's immunosuppression continued to deteriorate and candidal recurrences became more frequent, more severe, and less responsive.

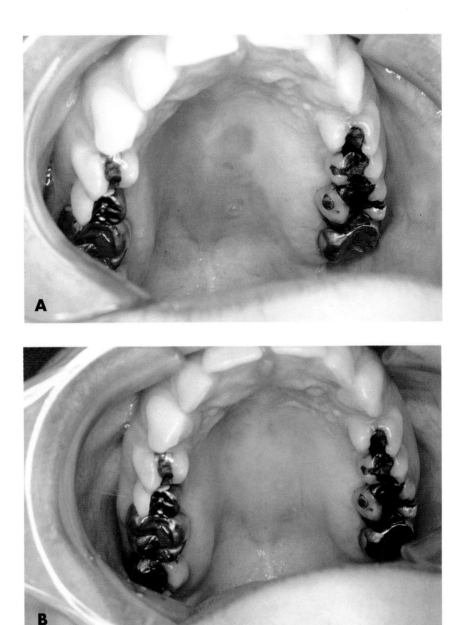

Figure 3.15 A, Painful erythematous candidal palatal infection in an otherwise asymptomatic HIV-positive gay man. **B,** Signs and symptoms disappeared after 1 week on topical antifungal medication.

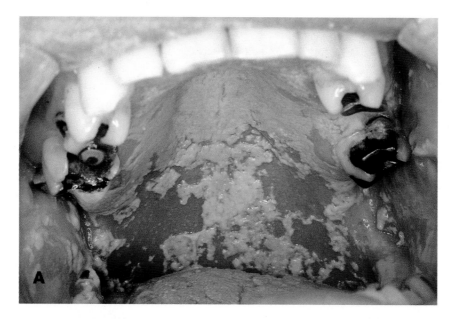

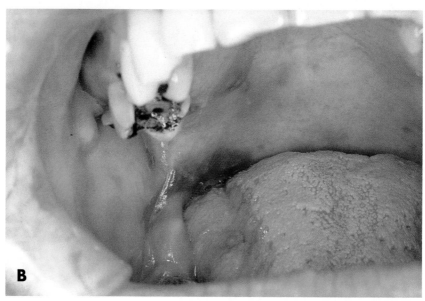

Figure 3.16 A, Florid candidiasis in a homosexual male who did not realize he was HIV-positive. This was his only complaint. **B,** Systemic antifungal medication cleared the candidal lesions. However, the underlying purple-red lesions were then observed and confirmed by biopsy as Kaposi's sarcoma. He obviously had AIDS and died 4 months later of *Pneumocystis carinii* pneumonia.

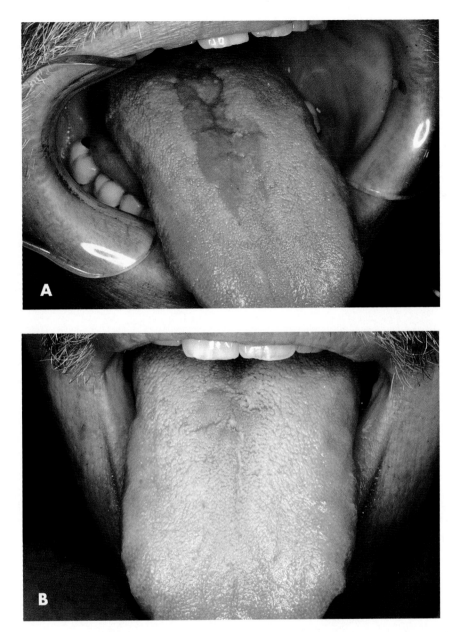

Figure 3.17 A, This otherwise asymptomatic gay male had a painful depapillated area on his tongue dorsum. A scraping showed candidiasis and a subsequent serology revealed HIV antibodies. **B,** Systemic antifungal medication reversed the signs and symptoms in 1 week.

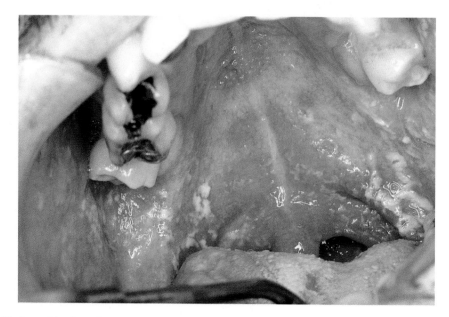

Figure 3.18 A combination of pseudomembranous and erythematous candidiasis in a heterosexual drug user, who had a rapidly decreasing CD4 count. Fungal "resistance" was evident, as increasing dosages of systemic antifungal medications were required to control signs and symptoms. Also, recurrences were rapid when either the dosages were tapered or topical agents were substituted.

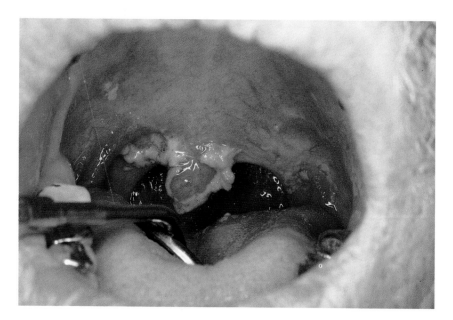

Figure 3.19 Hyperplastic candidiasis that could not be scraped off the mucosal surface. Cultures were *Candida*-positive, and the lesions disappeared in response to fluconazole 200 mg daily. The differential diagnosis had included leukoplakia with possible dysplasia or carcinoma. A biopsy was planned if the lesion had not responded to antifungal therapy.

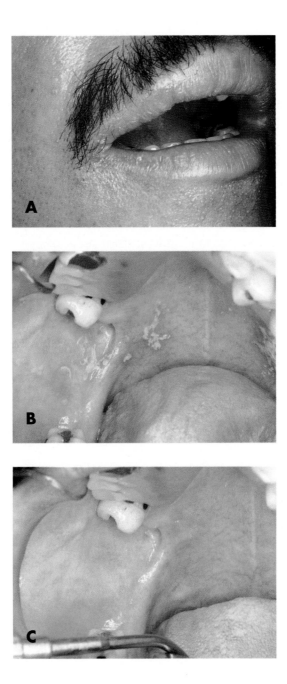

Figure 3-20 This 34-year-old asymptomatic gay man was seen for a routine oral examination as part of his health program. He was beginning to lose weight and felt "weak." Examination revealed angular cheilitis (**A**) and thrush (**B**). Response required 800 mg ketoconazole, indicating "resistance" over previously effective lower dosages (**C**). Recurrences were almost immediate, requiring chronic prophylaxis. His CD4 lymphocyte count was below 100. Megestrol (Megace) was prescribed to increase appetite and slow the progressive weight loss. He died 5 months after the acceleration of oral thrush.

HISTOPLASMOSIS

Histoplasma capsulatum is an opportunistic fungus that occurs endemically in various parts of the world, including the United States, and rarely infects the mouth. The infection is contracted by inhaling the airborne spores. Immunocompromised patients are at risk for disseminated disease, and as expected with HIV immunodeficiency, oral infections have been diagnosed, sometimes as the first sign of histoplasmosis. Because of varied signs and symptoms, the diagnosis of these lesions can be difficult. The diagnosis is established by biopsy, suspicious morphology, and immunoreactive stains.

Although the number of cases with oral manifestations is infrequent, it is apparent that the infections from histoplasmosis can occur at any oral mucosal site and usually present as an erosive or ulcerative lesion. Treatment entails a course of amphotericin B followed by prolonged oral antifungal drug intake. Unfortunately, oral manifestations are usually associated with systemic histoplasmosis and a declining CD4 count. Therefore overall prognosis is poor.

OTHER ORAL FUNGAL INFECTIONS

Oral manifestations caused by other fungi are extremely rare. Some of these fungal infections that may be associated with HIV immunosuppression include aspergillosis, cryptococcosis, geotrichosis, and mucormycosis. The oral lesions, when they occur, are usually associated with advanced AIDS patients who have little remaining immune competence. Clinical appearances are quite diverse, and diagnoses are established by biopsy and the use of special stains. Treatment often combines medical and surgical approaches.

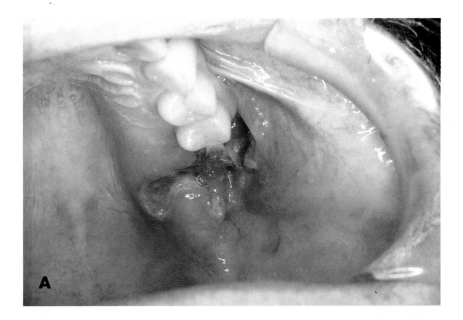

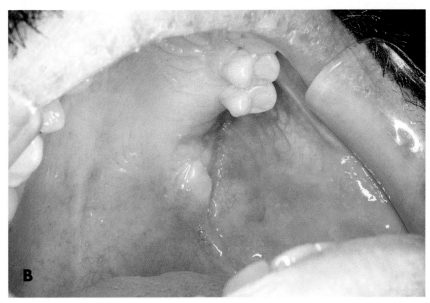

Figure 3.21 A, This 41-year-old heterosexual HIV-positive male was referred because of a painful and progressive gingival ulceration that had not responded to antibiotics and molar extractions. Differential diagnosis included progressive periodontal necrosis, lymphoma, or granulomatous disease. A biopsy confirmed a diagnosis of *Histoplasma capsulatum* infection. **B,** A 2-week hospital course of intravenous amphotericin B led to healing. Control was maintained with oral antifungals (ketoconazole) for 6 months. After discontinuation, he developed other opportunistic infections, including disseminated histoplasmosis.

SUGGESTED READINGS

Candidiasis: Clinical Features and Diagnosis

Duffy ED, Adelson R, Niessen LC, et al: VA Oral HIV Surveillance Program: Understanding the Disease. J Am Dent Assoc 1992; 123:57-62.

Hauman CHJ, Thompson IOC, Theunissen F, Wolfaardt P: Oral Carriage of *Candida* in Healthy and HIV-Seropositive Persons. Oral Surg Oral Med Oral Pathol 1993; 76:570-572.

Kirby AJ, Munoz A, Detels R, et al: Thrush and Fever as Measures of Immunocompetence in HIV-1-Infected Men. J Acquir Immun Defic Syndr 1994; 7:1242-1249.

Maden C, Hopkins SF, Lafferty WE: Progression to AIDS or Death Following Diagnosis with a Class IV Non-AIDS Disease: Utilization of a Surveillance Database. J Acquir Immun Defic Syndr 1994; 7:972-977.

McCarthy G: Host Factors Associated with HIV-Positive-Related Oral Candidiasis. Oral Surg Oral Med Oral Pathol 1992; 73:181-185.

Saah AJ, Hoover DR, He Y, et al: Factors Influencing Survival After AIDS: Report from the Multicenter AIDS Cohort Study (MACS). J Acquir Immun Defic Syndr 1994; 7:287-295.

Samaranayake L: Oral Mycoses in HIV Infection. Oral Surg Oral Med Oral Pathol 1992; 73:171-180.

Van Meter F, Gallo JW, Garcia-Rojas G, et al: A Study of Oral Candidiasis in HIV-Positive Patients. J Dent Hyg 1994; 68:30-34.

Candidiasis Treatment

Challacombe SJ: Immunologic Aspects of Oral Candidiasis. Oral Surg Oral Med Oral Pathol 1994; 78:202-210.

Como JA, Dismukes WE: Oral Azole Drugs as Systemic Antifungal Therapy. N Engl J Med 1994; 330:263-272.

Epstein JB, Burchell JL, Emerton S, et al: A Clinical Trial of Bethanechol in Patients with Xerostomia After Radiation Therapy. Oral Surg Oral Med Oral Pathol 1994; 77:610-614.

Miyasaki SH, Hicks JB, Greenspan D, et al: The Identification and Tracking of *Candida Albicans* Isolates from Oral Lesions in HIV-Seropositive Individuals. J Acquir Immun Defic Syndr 1992; 5:1039-1046.

Muzyka BC, Glick M: A Review of Oral Fungal Infections and Appropriate Therapy. J Am Dent Assoc 1995; 126: 63-72.

Odds FC: *Candida* Species and Virulence. ASM News 1994; 60:313-318.

Histoplasmosis

Chinn H, Chernoff DN, Migliorati CA, et al: Oral Histoplasmosis in HIV-Infected Patients. Oral Surg Oral Med Oral Pathol 1995; 79: 710-714.

Heinic GS, Greenspan D, MacPhail LA, et al: Oral *Histoplasma Capsulatum* Infection in Association with HIV Infection: A Case Report. J Oral Pathol Med 1992; 21:85-89.

Sarosi GA, Johnson PC: Disseminated Histoplasmosis in Patients Infected with Human Immunodeficiency Virus. Clin Infect Dis 1992; 14:560-567.

4 VIRAL INFECTIONS

Because HIV-infected individuals are immunocompromised, viral infections, which are opportunistic infections, occur more frequently and with greater severity. Some of these infections have long been known to occur in the oral cavity, but some others have been reported only since the outbreak of the AIDS epidemic. The increased prevalence produces more diverse clinical findings, often complicating diagnosis and management.

HIV protein rarely is found in the lesion, confirming the indirect effect of immunodeficiency as being the underlying cause of HIV-related pathology. These viral infections pose an increased threat to partners who may suffer also from immunodysregulation and susceptibility.

HERPES FAMILY VIRUSES

Herpes Simplex Virus-1 (HSV)

Herpes simplex virus-1 and sometimes HSV-2 are seen more frequently in HIV-infected individuals as compared to immunocompetent persons. The attacks are usually more severe, with recurrent lesions involving the lips (herpes labialis, "cold sores") and the oral mucosa. In both sites, lesions can persist for extended periods, they can be large, and they can occur as multiple ulcerations. Thus recognition can at times be difficult, leading to the use of wrong and ineffective therapeutic approaches.

When adults experience herpetic lip lesions for the first time or if attacks become more frequent and/or severe, immunosuppression should be suspected and included in the differential diagnosis. If a mucocutaneous herpetic flare is progressive and continues for more than 1 month in an HIV-positive patient, this condition meets the CDC criteria for an AIDS-defining disease. Intraoral recurrent herpes can occur on any mucosal surface, keratinized or unkeratinized, and can have quite diverse appearances of the ulcerative manifestations. Thus the differential diagnosis can be complex. There is almost always associated pain of varying degrees for both lip and mucosal sites.

The clinical diagnosis can be confused with toxic, allergic, and bacterial etiologies. When the clinical diagnosis is uncertain, the diagnosis can be confirmed by cultures to identify HSV, smears reacted with HSV-specific monoclonal antibodies, or cytologic scrapings to identify pseudogiant cells, which result from DNA proliferation without cell division. If a biopsy is obtained, HSV can be identified by morphologic cellular changes and immunoreactive stains.

Treatment depends on patient status and the severity (signs and symptoms) of the lesion(s). When there is evidence that a patient can still mount an immune response, management approaches can be by empirical supportive measures. Specific antiviral treatment involves the use of acyclovir (Zovirax). Because acyclovir is poorly absorbed and significant blood levels are required, daily dosages are high, ranging from 1 to 4 g.

Acyclovir itself is an inactive drug. It must be phosphorylated to the triphosphate form to be effective. This occurs in response to an enzyme, thymidine kinase, which is produced by the herpes virus. Acyclovir does not kill the virus; its effect is based on interference with DNA polymerase, temporarily stopping viral proliferation. Resistance to acyclovir takes place when HSV no longer produces thymidine kinase. Foscarnet (Foscavir) is an effective alternative antiviral drug, but it must be given intravenously. Topical antiviral ointments and creams have not been shown to be reproducibly helpful.

Recurrences are unpredictible, but expected. A prophylactic regimen can be useful, but effective dosages usually are determined on a trial-and-error basis, as are durations of treatment. Supportive measures should be instituted, including analgesic agents and adequate nutrition and hydration.

Herpes virus-6 has been of recent interest because of its occurrence in humans and some indications that it facilitates HIV infection of cells in vitro.

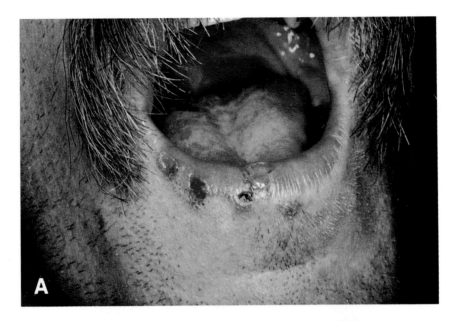

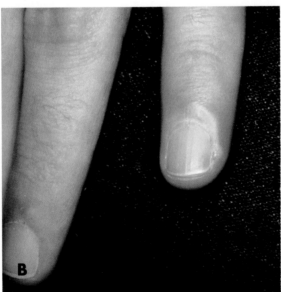

Figure 4.1 A, This 28-year-old homosexual male, who in the past had only occasional attacks of "cold sores," started manifesting multiple herpes labialis lesions that would continually recur. He was HIV-positive and was afflicted with other opportunistic infections. **B,** He was a nail biter and infected his nail beds with herpes simplex virus (herpetic whitlow).

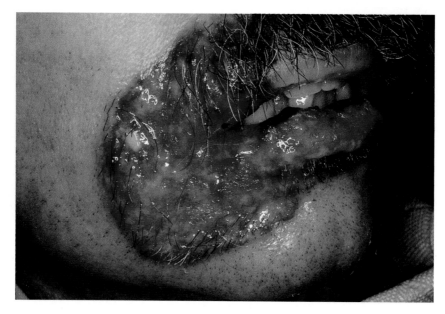

Figure 4.2 This HIV-positive patient had herpes labialis that was not self-limiting, and the infection spread to the adjacent skin. Mucocutaneous HSV infections that are progressive and persist for more than 1 month meet the CDC definition of AIDS in HIV-positive persons. Intravenous foscarnet was required for control.

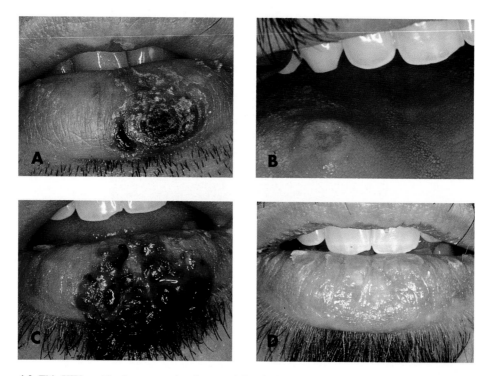

Figure 4.3 This HIV-positive homosexual male started developing cold sores that were much more severe and persisted for longer periods of time than he previously experienced. **A,** This herpetic lip lesion had persisted for 3 weeks. **B,** He also developed a lesion on the right dorsal tongue, which is typical for recurrent intraoral herpetic lesions in immunocompromised patients. It is commonly found in kidney transplant patients. **C,** At 4 weeks the lip lesion continued to extend and required treatment with acyclovir (1200 mg daily). **D,** After 10 days of treatment the lesion was brought under complete control.

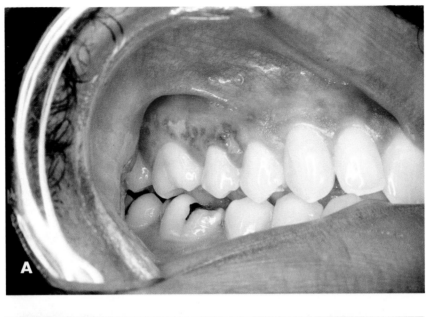

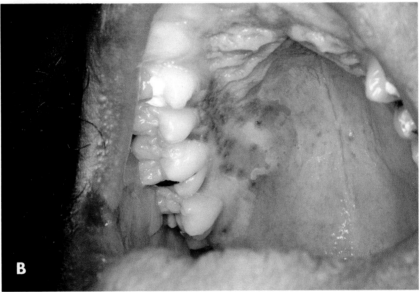

Figure 4.4 Recurrent intraoral herpetic lesions occur in nonimmunocompromised and immunocompromised patients. **A,** Recurrent HSV of gingiva. **B,** Recurrent HSV of palate.

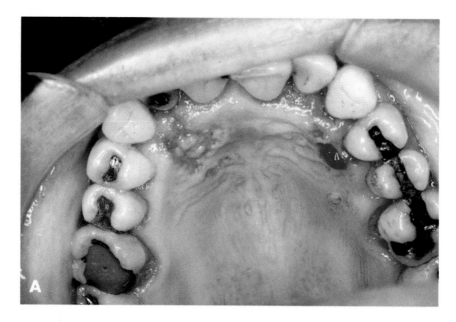

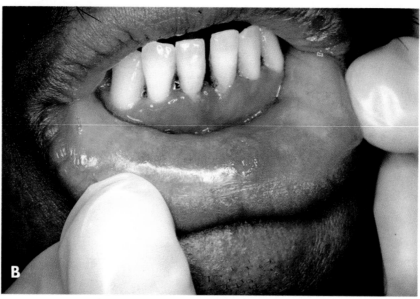

Figure 4.5 Recurrent herpes (HSV) of the palate in a 27-year-old HIV-positive gay male. **A,** The painful, hemorrhagic palatal lesions occurred in spite of low-dose acyclovir (400 mg/day) to control chronic genital herpes. **B,** The same patient also had an atypical-appearing ulcerative lesion of the lower labial unkeratinized mucosa that was shedding HSV. Note also the periodontal disease.

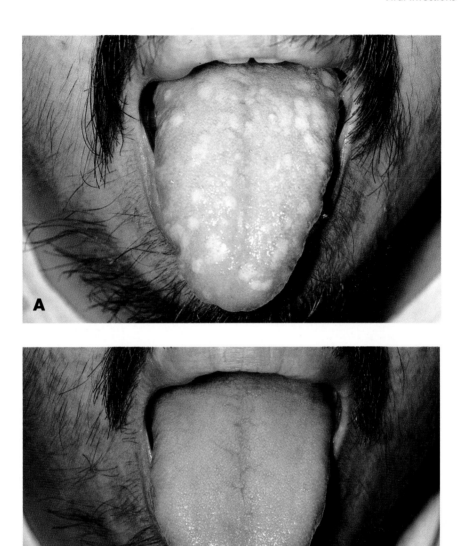

Figure 4.6 A, Atypical-appearing herpetic lesions (HSV) on the dorsum of the tongue of an HIV-positive hetero-sexual drug user. These painful lesions, which were HSV culture positive, had been present for 3 days, progres-sively worsening and precluding dietary intake. **B,** After 3 days of acyclovir (2 g daily), the lesions cleared as did the symptoms.

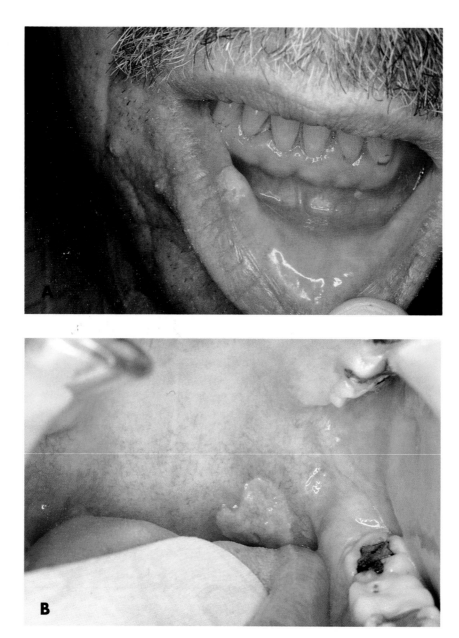

Figure 4.7 Recurrent intraoral herpes in immunocompromised patients can occur in any mucosal site. They often appear as pseudomembrane-covered mucosal erosions of irregular sizes and shapes. **A,** Recurrent HSV of labial mucosa. **B,** Recurrent HSV of soft palate.

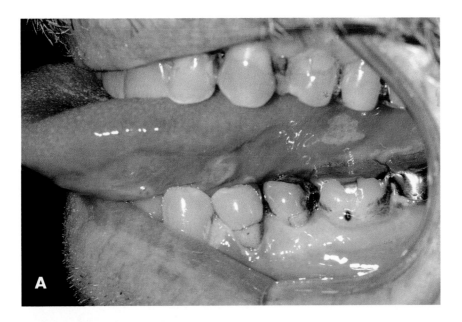

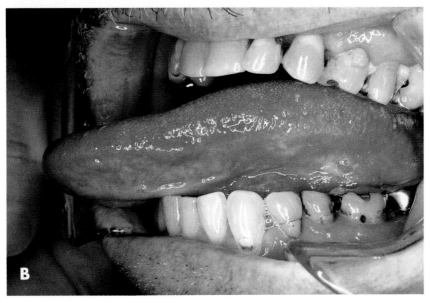

Figure 4.8 Recurrent HSV usually responds quite well to acyclovir in daily dosages exceeding 1 g. This treatment is usually effective until the terminal stages of AIDS. **A,** Increasing painful HSV lesions of the tongue that persisted over 2 weeks in a 32-year-old HIV-positive man. **B,** Signs and symptoms rapidly disappeared after 4 days of systemic acyclovir (1200 mg daily).

Epstein-Barr Virus (EBV) and Oral Hairy Leukoplakia (OHL)

EBV might well be a co-factor in several HIV-associated oral lesions. The most common is the association between EBV and OHL. OHL is almost always found unilaterally or bilaterally on the lateral border of the tongue. It usually presents as a corrugated or hair-like white lesion that can appear at times as flat white patches. Occasionally, OHL can occur on another oral mucosal surface. The extent of OHL is not necessarily correlated with the stage of HIV infection. In fact, OHL can be the first sign of HIV infection in some patients.

A clinician must be careful in establishing the diagnosis, since similar-appearing changes can occur in HIV-negative persons. Some examples include lichen planus, leukoplakia, candidiasis, immunosuppression secondary to chemotherapy, and irritational keratoses. OHL is not related to precancerous leukoplakia or dysplasias.

When uncertainties exist or more information is needed for management, the diagnosis is established by biopsy to identify tissue patterns and EBV. Characteristic features include epithelial hyperplasia, immature surface keratin (no keratohyaline granules), vacuolated squamous cells (koilocytes), and variable to no connective tissue inflammation. When required to further confirm the diagnosis, EBV can be detected using in situ hybridization and special DNA probes. Cytologic smears from OHL will frequently reveal pathognomonic margination and clumping of nuclear protein.

OHL primarily occurs in homosexual and bisexual men, although it has been reported in other HIV-afflicted groups. This suggests some other unidentified co-factor(s) that may well be transmitted most efficiently by anal sex. While EBV is associated with OHL, its exact role in the etiology and transmission is not clear. Absence of Langerhans cells and altered mucosal immunity seem to play roles also.

If a patient does not know his/her HIV status, OHL mandates HIV testing. OHL is rarely symptomatic. Since there is no clearcut relationship between removing OHL and either quality of life or survival, treatment is elective and usually on the basis of a patient complaint that the lesion is "bothersome."

Many different approaches will temporarily control OHL, but once a treatment is discontinued, OHL will sooner or later recur. Successful temporary control has been obtained using antivirals in high dosages (acyclovir), starting AZT antiretroviral therapy, in patients who are being simultaneously treated with trimethoprim-sulfamethoxazole (Bactrim or Septra) for pneumocystic pneumonia, topical application of 0.05% Retin A solution, and topical application of keratinolytic podophyllin (25% solution in tincture of benzoin).

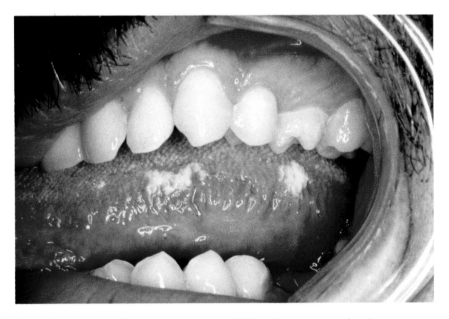

Figure 4.9 Limited hairy leukoplakia in an asymptomatic HIV-positive homosexual male.

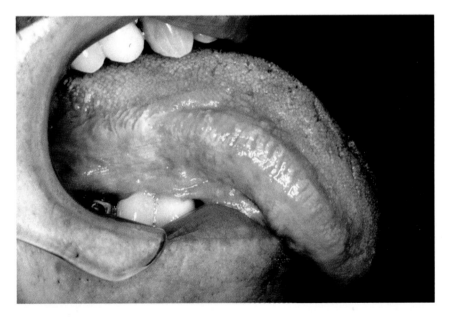

Figure 4.10 Limited asymptomatic hairy leukoplakia in a 30-year-old homosexual male. He was otherwise in apparent good health; this was the first sign of HIV infection.

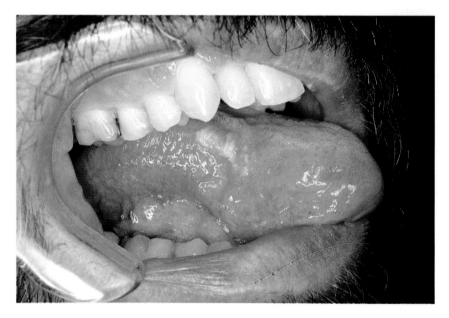

Figure 4.11 Asymptomatic limited hairy leukoplakia.

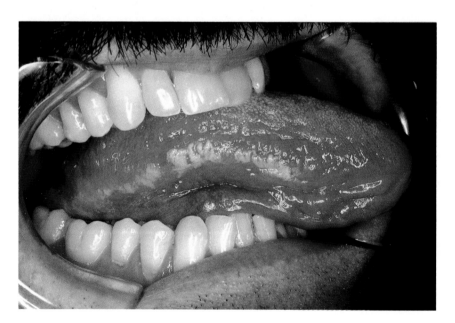

Figure 4.12 A more typical appearance of hairy leukoplakia, demonstrating the corrugated and hair-like appearance that prompted the name.

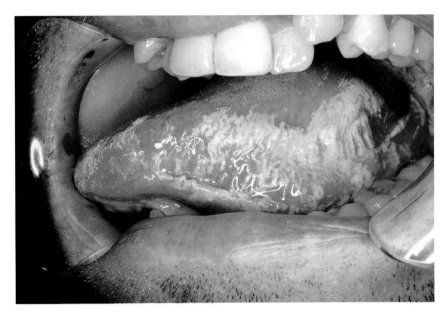

Figure 4.13 A more extensive hairy leukoplakia in a 30-year-old HIV-positive homosexual male. He also had oropharyngeal candidiasis; however, the oral candidiasis responded to antifungal treatment, while the hairy leukoplakia lesion remained. It was essentially asymptomatic.

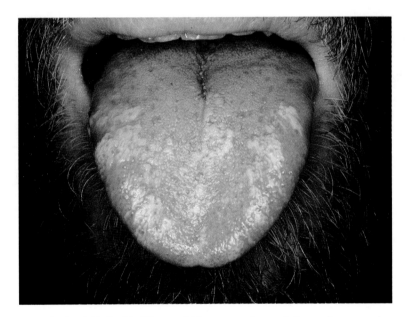

Figure 4.14 The hairy leukoplakia in this 27-year-old homosexual extended onto the tongue dorsum. Except for a mild chronic candidiasis, the patient was without any other signs or symptoms. Six months later he developed *Pneumocystis carinii* pneumonia.

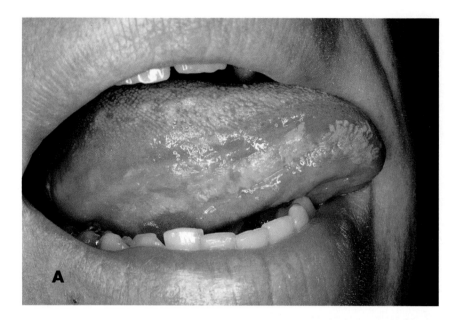

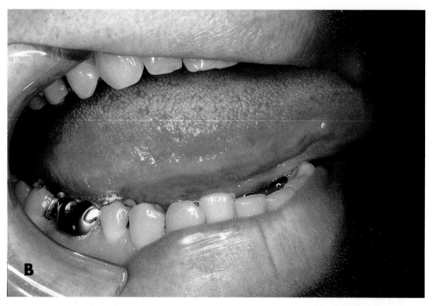

Figure 4.15 Treatment of hairy leukoplakia is nonspecific and elective. **A,** Mildly symptomatic hairy leukoplakia. The patient also had pneumocystic pneumonia and was put on azidothymidine (AZT). **B,** After 1 month on daily AZT, and without any other forms of management, the hairy leukoplakia essentially disappeared clinically.

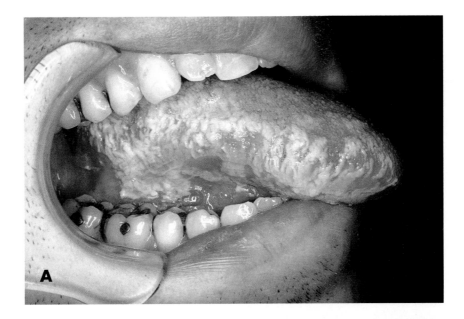

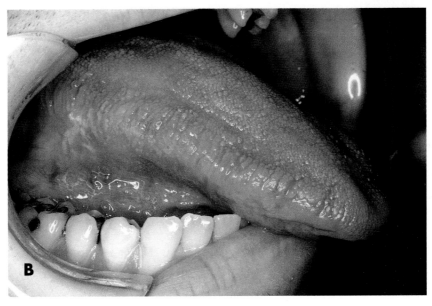

Figure 4.16 Most hairy leukoplakias will go into clinical remission on large doses of acyclovir. **A,** Pretreatment appearance. **B,** Appearance following 2 g of daily acyclovir for 2 weeks. When the acyclovir was discontinued, the lesion slowly returned to the same site and extent.

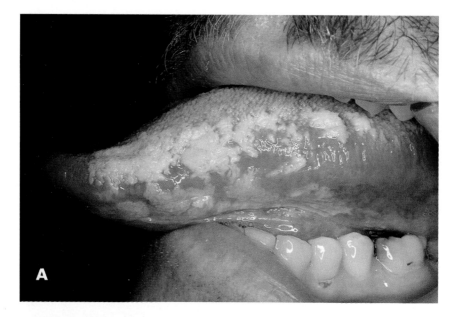

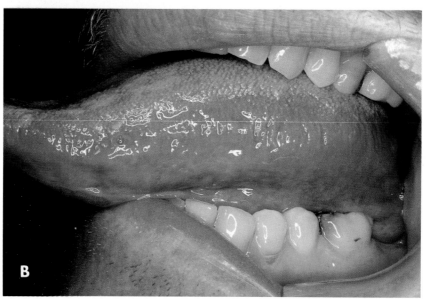

Figure 4.17 This 34-year-old HIV-infected homosexual man had been stable for 6 years with a CD4 count of 260, oral hairy leukoplakia (OHL), and occasional thrush. **A,** The OHL started to become more prominent and "irritating." A 30-second application of 25% podophyllin was applied in the clinic. **B,** One week later, without any changes in medications, habits, or food patterns, he was without signs or symptoms. The control from the treatment lasted 3 months.

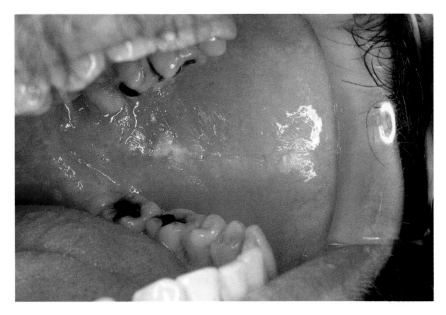

Figure 4.18 Hairy leukoplakia occasionally will occur on sites other than the lateral borders of the tongue. This 32-year-old HIV-positive homosexual male had biopsy-proven hairy leukoplakia on the buccal mucosa as well as the tongue.

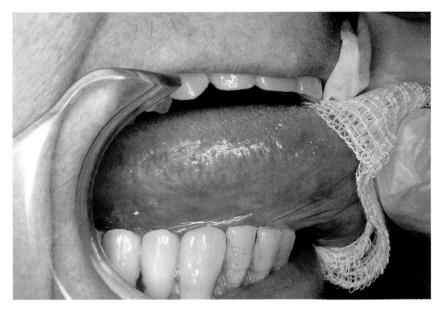

Figure 4.19 Many lesions may resemble hairy leukoplakia. Because of the significance regarding HIV infection implied by hairy leukoplakia, clinical suspicion must be confirmed. This patient, who was concerned about being immunocompromised, had biopsy-proven lichen planus. A subsequent serology showed her to be HIV-negative.

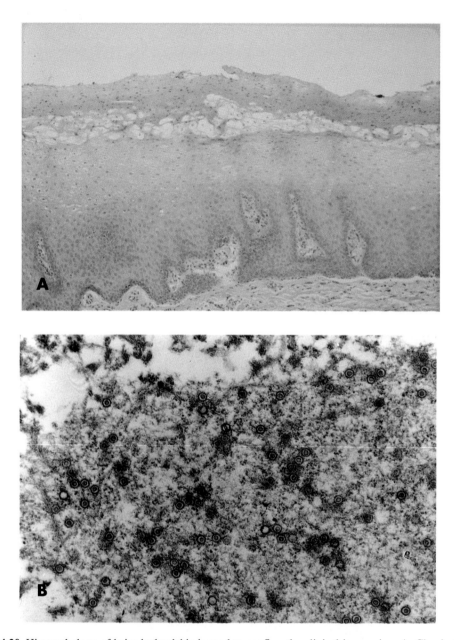

Figure 4.20 Histopathology of hairy leukoplakia is used to confirm the clinical impression. **A,** Classical appearance of hairy leukoplakia, demonstrating epithelial hyperplasia, little or no connective tissue inflammation, a pseudokeratin surface layer, and multiple vacuolated cells associated with Epstein-Barr virus infection. The vacuolated cells have been referred to as koilocytes, implying viral infection. **B,** An electron microscopic photomicrograph of part of a nucleus of a vacuolated cell, demonstrating Epstein-Barr viruses interspersed in the nuclear protein.

Varicella Virus Reactivation (Zoster, Shingles)

In the immunocompromised patient, the risk exists for reactivation of latent chickenpox virus. When this happens, the disease takes the form of varicella zoster, more commonly referred to as herpes zoster or shingles. The vesicles formed by the virus eventually break and scab or are covered by pseudomembranes. Zoster lesions present a classical unilateral pattern and are associated with both pruritus and pain. They can become secondarily infected.

While the lesions are usually self-limiting, the most important symptoms are the postzoster neuropathy and pain which can be excruciating. Therefore high-dose acyclovir treatment is instituted (e.g., 800 mg every 5 to 6 hours). Simultaneous high-dose prednisone may be helpful. Control of fever and pain as well as adequate nutrition and hydration are important in the treatment. Famciclovir is a more recent antiviral drug that has been useful for acute zoster (500 mg three times daily). Recurrences are uncommon. However, the occurrence of zoster in the HIV patient often indicates advanced staging, development of other opportunistic infections, and a poor prognosis for lengthy survival.

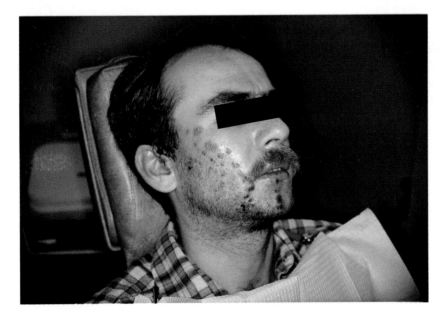

Figure 4.21 This HIV-positive patient experienced reactivation of his latent varicella (chickenpox) virus and acutely developed right facial pruritus, fever, and malaise, Three days later, vesicles and scabbed ulcers were evident in a typical unilateral zoster distribution. The attack signaled a declining CD4 count, and the patient subsequently died from other opportunistic infections.

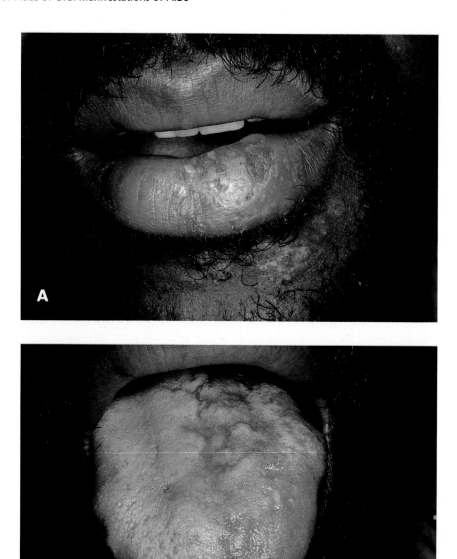

Figure 4.22 A, This HIV-positive Afro-American presented because of painful ulcerations on the left chin, vermilion border, and tongue dorsum. **B,** A clinical diagnosis of varicella zoster (shingles) was made and the patient was started on supportive care of analgesics, antipyretics, and nutritional support. His condition cleared in 10 days, but he experienced postzoster neuropathic pain. Following the attack, he developed the wasting syndrome (unintentional weight loss), which was concomitant with a falling CD4 count.

Cytomegalovirus (CMV)

CMV antibodies are found in over 50% of the normal population, indicating the frequency of human exposure to this virus. Antibodies to CMV can almost always be found in patients made immunodeficient with HIV, and frequently the virus itself can be cultivated. In the HIV-positive patient, CMV can cause many debilitating conditions. The most common is CMV retinitis, which may even lead to blindness.

While oral lesions due to CMV are rarely reported, this might be due to difficulties in establishing the diagnosis. They usually present as nonspecific ulcers that can be mistaken for other infections, granulomatous lesions, inflammatory/immunologic diseases, or malignancies. Pain is the common complaint. Diagnosis is established by biopsy, recognition of suggestive microscopic morphologic changes (e.g., "owl-eye cells"), and the use of immunoreactive stains.

CMV may also serve as a co-factor in salivary gland enlargement and hypofunction leading to xerostomia. Therefore the role of CMV in many HIV-associated conditions has yet to be completely clarified. CMV may even be a co-factor in HIV progression. In any event, the antiviral drug ganciclovir (Cytovene) has been selectively effective in controlling CMV infections.

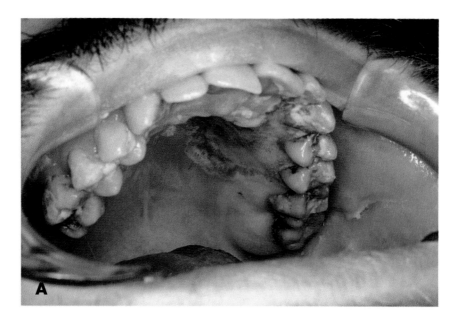

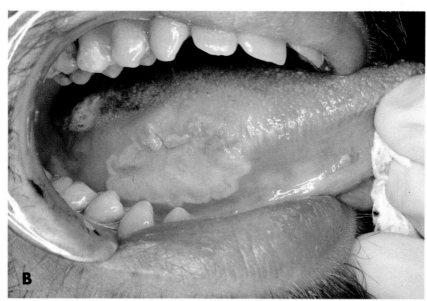

Figure 4.23 This 36-year-old homosexual male was referred because of excruciating pain in the palate and tongue, extending to the esophagus. His CD4 count was less than 100. The complaints were now into the fifth week and worsening. Antifungal and antibiotic courses did not help. The severe symptoms precluded eating, and the patient was progressively losing weight and becoming psychologically depressed. Clinical examination revealed a necrotic, cavernous ulcer of the palate (**A**) and an extensive pseudomembrane-covered ulceration of the tongue (**B**).

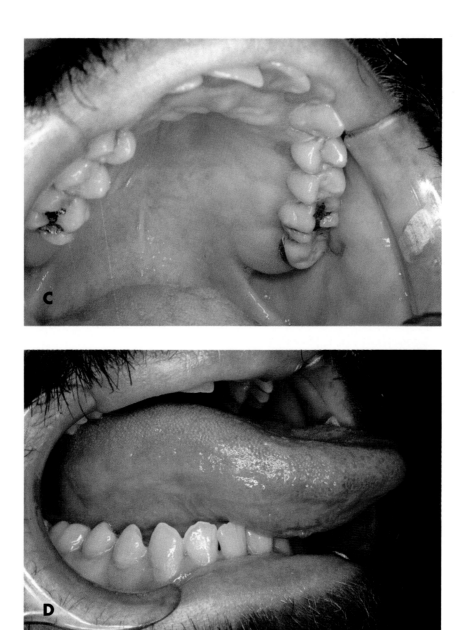

Figure 4.23—cont'd. A biopsy from each lesion showed a mixed viral infection of connective tissue cytomegalovirus and epithelial herpes virus. A course of ganciclovir (Cytovene) was started, and within 3 weeks the ulcers had healed (**C** and **D**), all symptoms disappeared, a normal diet was taken, and his weight stabilized.

HUMAN PAPILLOMAVIRUS (HPV) AND CONDYLOMA ACUMINATUM

The presence of HPV is so common in oral mucosa that the significance of being causal, co-factor, or passenger is difficult to document. However, certain strains are known to be related to condylomata acuminata (venereal warts) and their increased occurrence in HIV patients. This is due to an increase in unprotected sex as well as immunosuppression. Often these individuals also manifest genital and anal condylomata. When the strain is HPV-16, the infection risks are associated with the development of squamous carcinomas (anus, uterine cervix). In HIV-positive women, carcinoma of the cervix is an AIDS-defining disease.

The diagnosis of oral condyloma can usually be made by appearance and history. While they primarily appear as verruca, the lesions can be somewhat flat and smooth, resembling fibromas. Biopsy and appropriate probes or PCR techniques can establish HPV presence and strain.

Treatment of oral lesions involves tissue removal of significant depth to remove all localized virus. Electrosurgical and laser techniques are well suited for these procedures. Since reinfection is common, control of warts at other sites and counseling regarding infected partners are essential. While condylomata are not necessarily consistent with HIV infection, because of similar high-risk behavior a possible association must be presumed until ruled out.

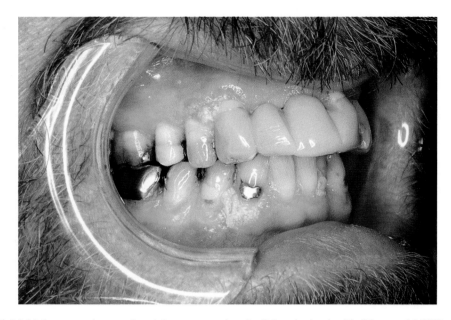

Figure 4.24 Multiple venereal warts (condylomata acuminata) of the gingiva in this 34-year-old HIV-positive homosexual man.

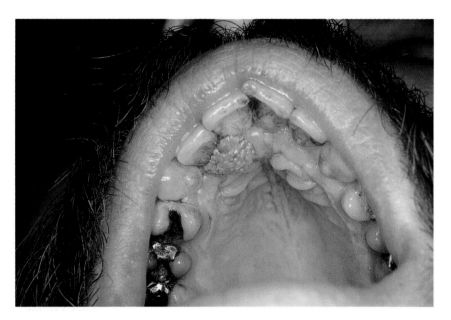

Figure 4.25 A large venereal wart in an HIV-positive homosexual male, who also has venereal warts on the genitalia.

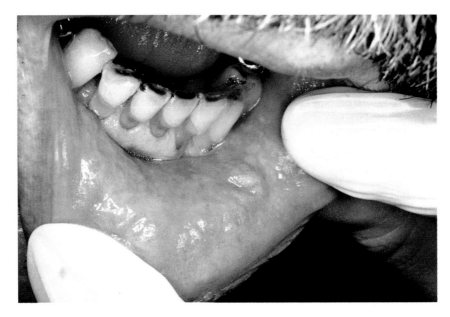

Figure 4.26 Venereal wart of the lower lip in a sexually active HIV-positive homosexual man.

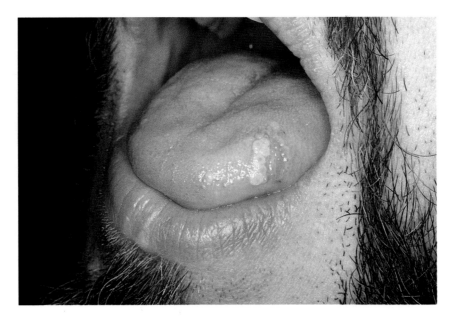

Figure 4.27 Venereal wart of the tongue that was mildly bothersome to the patient. This HIV-positive man also had anal condylomata.

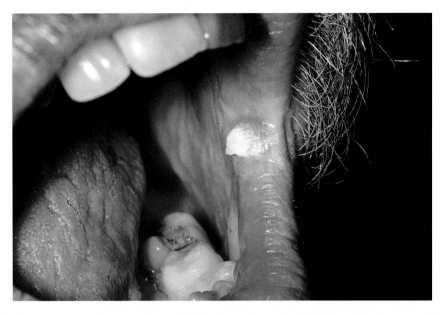

Figure 4.28 A large symptomatic venereal wart of the left commissure in this HIV-positive homosexual male.

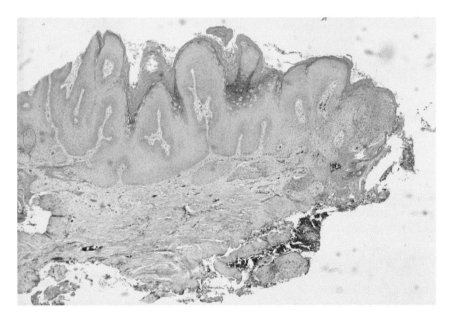

Figure 4.29 Classical histologic presentation of a venereal wart, demonstrating irregular epithelial hyperplasia, hyperkeratosis, and vacuolated epithelial cells that are infected with various strains of human papillomavirus.

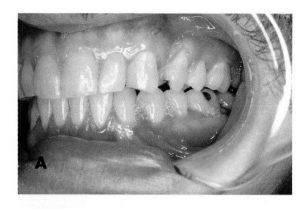

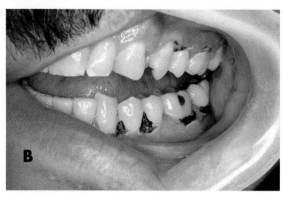

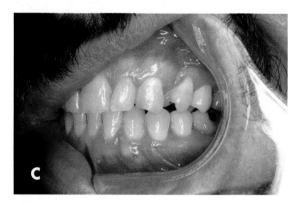

Figure 4.30 A, This 30-year-old HIV-positive bisexual man presented with asymptomatic condylomata acuminata (venereal warts) of the gingiva. He had multiple partners and was an occasional drug user. **B,** All observed lesions were removed by carbon dioxide laser. **C,** Healing was complete in 10 days.

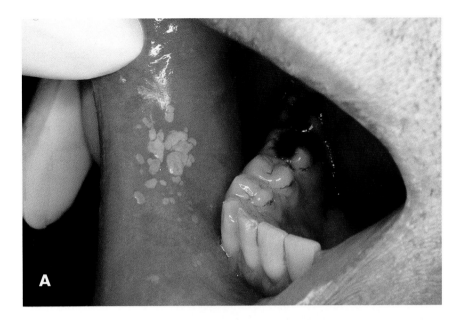

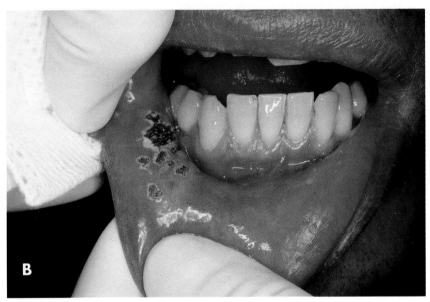

Figure 4.31 A, Condylomata can appear as flat, smooth, slightly keratotic lesions that resemble fibromas. These were removed using a laser **(B)**. This patient was HIV-positive and had a history of previous venereal warts in the mouth and genital area. Recurrences are common from self-infection and infected partners.

MOLLUSCUM CONTAGIOSUM (MC)

Molluscum contagiosum (MC) is a DNA virus of the poxvirus family. While intraoral lesions are extremely rare, facial skin lesions are not too uncommon in HIV-immunocompromised patients. The lesions occur as papules that can burst and become secondarily infected. MC is of concern because of appearance, discomfort, and the possibility of spread by direct contact. There is no reproducibly effective treatment.

HEPATITIS VIRUSES

No specific oral lesions are associated with hepatitis viruses. However, because of the virulence and transmission risks of hepatitis viruses B (HBV) and C (HCV, previously non-A, non-B) and similar modes of transmission with HIV, these viruses are of significance to clinicians.

Because of improved acceptance and use of barrier techniques and sterilization methods, there have been no reported cases of transmission from HBV-positive dentists to dental patients since 1987. Conversely, following the large acceptance of the effective HBV vaccine, HBV infection has not been a significant threat to practitioners. However, with the now known diversity of transmission of HCV (similar to HBV) and the lack of a vaccine, a possible risk remains. HCV infection is associated with increased sickness and greater risk for chronic hepatitis. Two other hepatitis strains are now recognized: the more often fatal D, which requires HBV antigen for infection, and E.

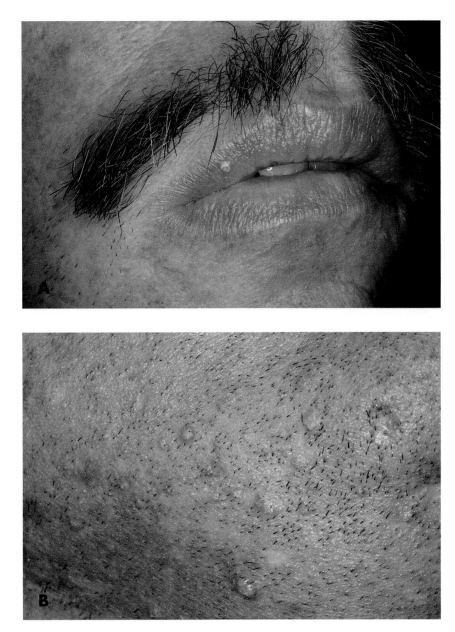

Figure 4.32 HIV-associated lesions of molluscum contagiosum. Note typical manifestations from this virus on the upper right vermilion border (**A**) and pustular papules on facial skin (**B**).

SUGGESTED READINGS

Herpes Simplex Virus

Agut H: Puzzles Concerning the Pathogenicity of Human Herpesvirus 6. N Engl J Med 1993; 329:293-294.

Balfour HH Jr, Benson C, Braun J, et al: Management of Acyclovir-Resistant Herpes Simplex and Varicella-Zoster Virus Infections. J Acquir Immun Defic Syndr 1994; 7:254- 260.

Epstein JB, Rea G, Sibau L, Sherlock CH: Rotary Dental Instruments and the Potential Risk of Transmission of Infection: Herpes Simplex Virus. J Am Dent Assoc 1993; 123:55-59.

Eversole LR: Viral Infections of the Head and Neck Among HIV-Seropositive Patients. Oral Surg Oral Med Oral Pathol 1992; 73:155-163.

Hall CB, Long CE, Schnabel KC, et al: Human Herpesvirus-6 Infection in Children. N Engl J Med 1994; 331:432-438.

Miller CS, Redding SW: Diagnosis and Management of Orofacial Herpes Simplex Virus Infections. Dent Clin N Am 1992; 36:879-895.

Oral Hairy Leukoplakia

Greenspan D, Greenspan JS: Significance of Oral Hairy Leukoplakia. Oral Surg Oral Med Oral Pathol 1992; 73:151- 154.

Lozada-Nur F, Robinson J, Regezi JA: Oral Hairy Leukoplakia in Nonimmunosuppressed Patients. Report of Four Cases. Oral Surg Oral Med Oral Pathol 1994; 78:599-602.

Pagano JS: Epstein-Barr Virus: Culprit or Consort? N Engl J Med 1992; 327:1750-1752.

Schmidt M, Norgaard T, Greenspan JS: Oral Hairy Leukoplakia in an HIV-Negative Woman With Behcet's Syndrome. Oral Surg Oral Med Oral Pathol 1995; 79:53-56.

Varicella Virus and Zoster

Gilden DH: Herpes Zoster with Postherpetic Neuralgia—Persisting Pain and Frustration. N Engl J Med 1994; 330:932- 933.

Wood MJ, Johnson RW, McKendrick MW, et al: A Randomized Trial of Acyclovir for 7 Days or 21 Days With and Without Prednisolone for Treatment of Acute Herpes Zoster. N Engl J Med 1994; 330:896-900.

Cytomegalovirus

Epstein JB, Sherlock CH, Wolber RA: Oral Manifestations of Cytomegalovirus Infection. Oral Surg Oral Med Oral Pathol 1993; 75:443-451.

Greenberg MS, Dubin G, Stewart JCB, et al: Relationship of Oral Disease to the Presence of Cytomegalovirus DNA in the Saliva of AIDS Patients. Oral Surg Oral Med Oral Pathol 1995; 79: 175-179.

Jones AC, Freedman PD, Phelan JA, et al: Cytomegalovirus Infection of the Oral Cavity: A Report of Six Cases and Review of the Literature. Oral Surg Oral Med Oral Pathol 1993; 75:76-85.

Webster A: Cytomegalovirus as a Possible Cofactor in HIV Disease Progression. J Aquir Immun Defic Syndr 1991; 4(Suppl. 1):S47-S52.

Human Papillomavirus

Zuess MS, Miller CS, White DK: In Situ Hybridization Analysis of Human Papillomavirus DNA in Oral Mucosal Lesions. Oral Surg Oral Med Oral Pathol 1991; 71:714-720.

Hepatitis Viruses

Alter MJ, Margolis HS, Krawczynski K, et al: The Natural History of Community-Acquired Hepatitis C in the United States. N Engl J Med 1992; 327:1899-1905.

Porter S, Scully C, Samaranayake L: Viral Hepatitis: Current Concepts for Dental Practice. Oral Surg Oral Med Oral Pathol 1994; 78;682-695.

5

BACTERIAL INFECTIONS

NECROTIZING ULCERATIVE GINGIVITIS/PERIODONTITIS

The frequent occurrence of unusual and unexpected gingivitis and periodontitis in HIV-infected patients confirms an association between immunosuppression and these inflammatory/infectious conditions. This consequence of HIV disease is not surprising based on the loss of protective salivary enzymes, some changes in the subgingival microbial flora, suppressed responses of tissue immune components, and altered leukocyte functions. This involvement can be acute and often is progressive, causing pain and leading to exposed, necrotic bone and tooth mobility. In the chronic form, gingival inflammation and necrosis with subsequent destruction of alveolar bone can progress rather rapidly.

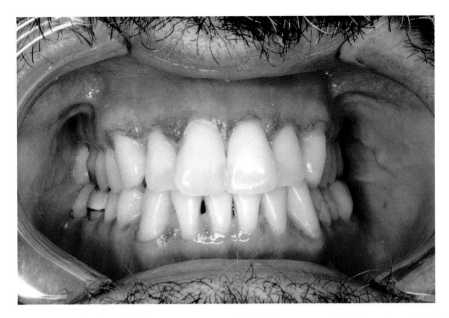

Figure 5.1 Speckled, telangiectatic-like asymptomatic gingivitis was one of the first signs of HIV infection. Although this patient was *Candida*-positive, the gingival lesions remained after antifungal treatment and a subsequent negative culture. The gingivitis was also nonresponsive to antibiotics. Blood counts were normal, as were platelets. A biopsy revealed a nonspecific "mucositis."

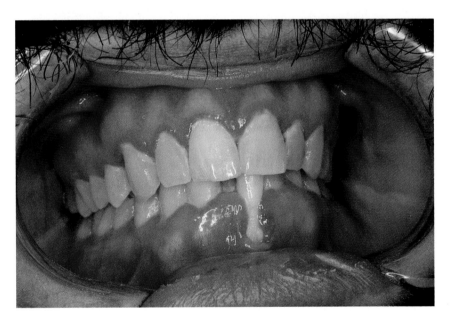

Figure 5.2 Gingivitis was the first marker in this HIV-infected patient. Note the severe gingival clefting involving the lower central incisor. The inflammatory change seen in the maxillary gingiva is often referred to as linear marginal erythema.

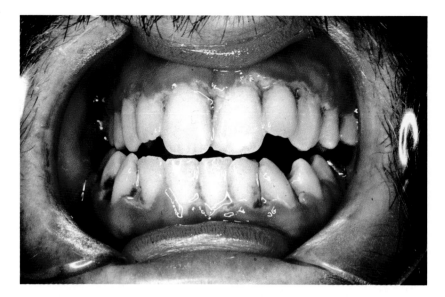

Figure 5.3 Commonly seen subacute necrotizing ulcerative gingivitis in a 32-year-old HIV-positive patient. It is often progressive and required aggressive treatment.

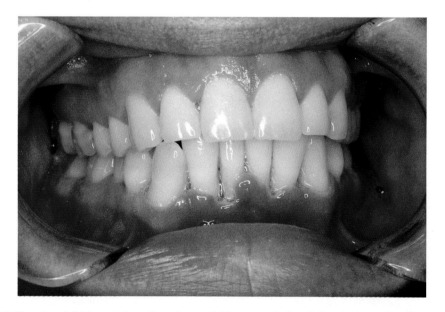

Figure 5.4 Chronic painful necrotizing, ulcerative gingivitis, and periodontal disease in an otherwise asymptomatic HIV-infected 30-year-old patient.

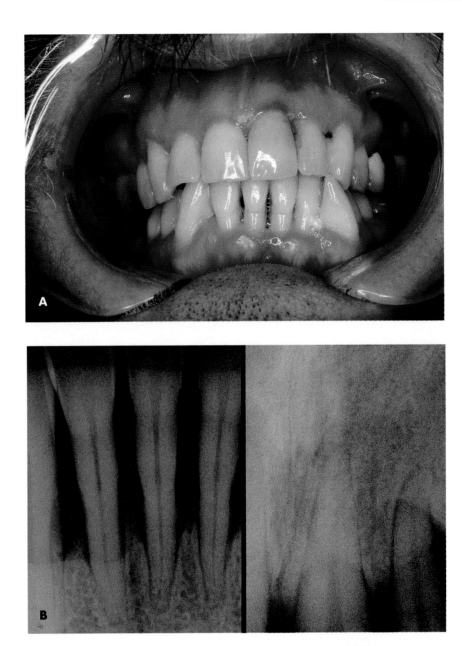

Figure 5.5 A, Progressive gingival recession and alveolar bone resorption in an AIDS patient. Note vascular-like lesion associated with the marginal gingiva of the upper left central incisor. A biopsy of the maxillary lesion proved to be Kaposi's sarcoma and the first sign of AIDS. **B,** Note radiographic evidence of loss of bone.

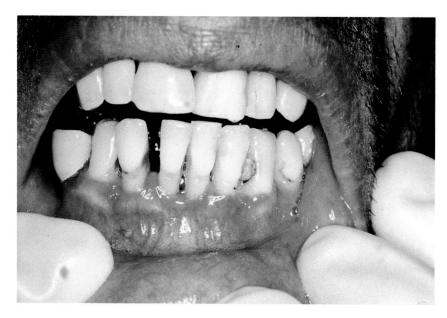

Figure 5.6 Advanced and progressive periodontal disease in a 34-year-old male with AIDS.

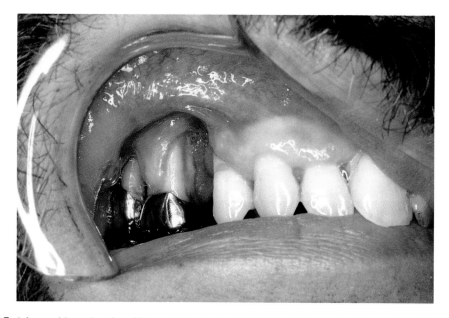

Figure 5.7 Advanced bone loss in a 29-year-old patient with AIDS-related complex. Aggressive office and home care, including the use of antibiotics, was not able to control this progressive infection.

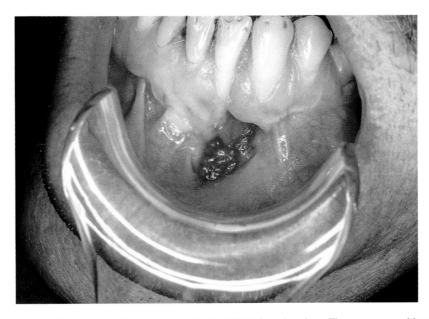

Figure 5.8 An area of mucosal and bone necrosis in the HIV-infected patient. There was no evident cause, and response to management regimens was slow.

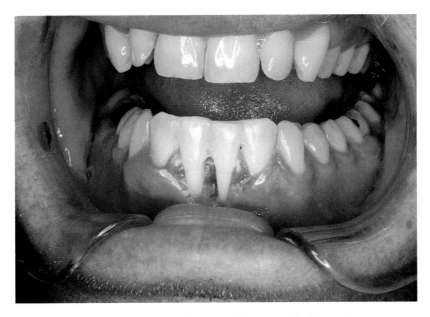

Figure 5.9 This 39-year-old gay man was referred because of the unexplainable gingival recession associated with his two lower central incisors. He had no other complaints or findings. Splinting and curettage had not controlled the progression. Biopsy of the interdental granulomatous tissue showed only nonspecific inflammation. The patient agreed to HIV testing to determine the possibility of immunosuppression. He was HIV-positive and a CD4 lymphocyte count was 340 (normal >700).

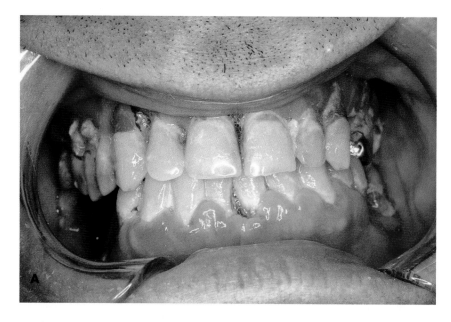

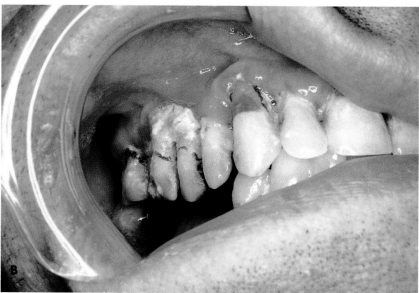

Figure 5.10 A, This 30-year-old HIV-positive drug abuser with extremely poor hygiene had progressive periodontal disease. **B,** Note the osteonecrosis involving the upper right posterior quadrant. Temporary control was achieved by curettage, home care compliance, antibiotics, and a disinfectant mouth rinse.

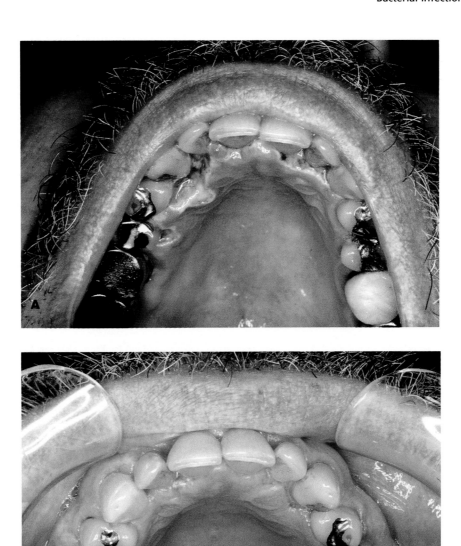

Figure 5.11 A, Acute necrotizing ulcerative gingivitis in a 36-year-old AIDS patient. T4-lymphocytes approximated 200 cells/mm^3 blood. **B,** Ten days of metronidazole (1000 mg/day) with amoxicillin (1500 mg/day) and a chlorhexidine mouth rinse induced healing.

The diagnosis is based on history and radiographic and clinical findings. Spontaneous bleeding, or bleeding on probing, is not unusual. This finding can be exaggerated in some HIV patients who also may be suffering from thrombocytopenia (low platelet count). The gingiva may manifest an idiopathic marginal linear erythema or a generalized erythema. In the latter case, candidiasis must be considered in the differential diagnosis.

Treatment requires an aggressive program of home and office care, simultaneously recognizing the importance of long-term maintenance. When indicated, debridement should be instituted. Use of antiseptic mouth rinses, like 0.12% chlorhexidine (Peridex, PerioGard), is a must to supplement routine professional office management and conscientious home care. Antibiotics are frequently required. Suggestions include metronidazole (Flagyl, 1000 mg daily), combined, based on judgment, with a gram-positive antibiotic, such as amoxicillin (1500 mg daily); or a broad spectrum bactericidal antibiotic such as clindamycin (Clindacin, 900 to 1200 mg daily). Many times, extraction is the optimal therapeutic choice. Compliance is often a problem based on depression, forgetfulness, costs, social problems, and other HIV-associated sickness.

NON-ORAL-FLORA OPPORTUNISTS

Bacteria not ordinarily found as part of the oral flora can cause opportunistic mouth infections in the immunodeficient patient. Fortunately, this condition is not commonly found, recognized, or reported. The most common causative agents arise from the respiratory and gastrointestinal tracts, as example, *Klebsiella pneumoniae* (respiratory) and *Escherichia coli* (gastrointestinal).

Management entails suspicion of an infectious source and performing a culture if there is no response to usual care.

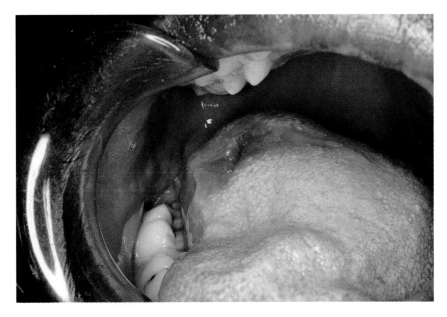

Figure 5.12 This 25-year-old HIV-positive man presented with a painful, indurated, ulcerative mass of his right tongue. It had been present for 1 month and was thought to represent a malignancy. A biopsy showed no tumor (nonspecific inflammation only). A culture taken at the time of biopsy revealed an almost pure growth of *E. coli*. A 10-day course of clindamycin (1200 mg daily) led to complete remission of signs and symptoms.

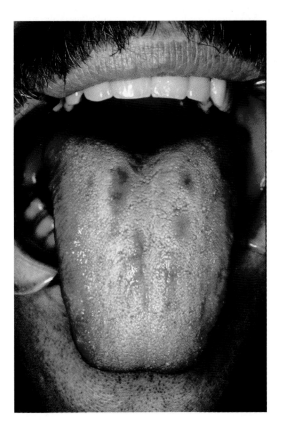

Figure 5.13 *Klebsiella pneumoniae* infection of the tongue causing painful, erythematous lesions that responded to antibiotic therapy. The diagnosis was suspected from culture results.

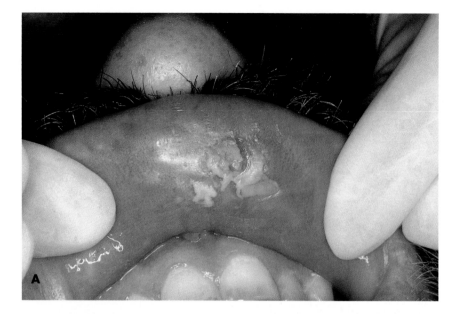

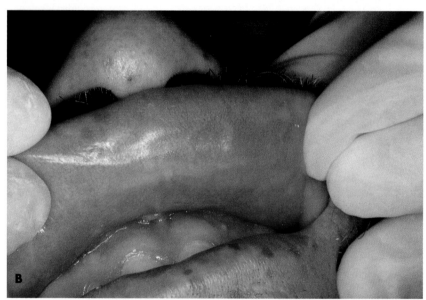

Figure 5.14 A, This indurated ulcerative lesion had been present for 2 weeks in this HIV-positive patient, who had multiple sex partners. An RPR (rapid plasma reagin) test, which measures nonspecific antibodies of syphilis, was positive. **B,** High-dose penicillin was initiated and 1 week later the ulcer had healed and was asymptomatic. The lesion was assumed to be a mucosal manifestation of secondary syphilis.

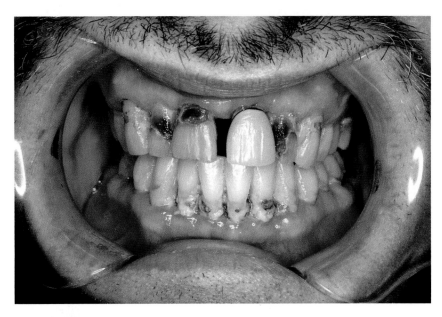

Figure 5.15 This HIV-positive drug user, age 25, reported with rampant caries and progressive periodontal disease. Possible explanations of this not infrequent finding include neglect and poor hygiene, alterations in the oral flora, and quantitative/qualitative salivary changes.

TUBERCULOSIS (TB)

TB very rarely will cause an oral lesion, but like hepatitis, it creates a risk to health care professional workers. In recent years, TB has increased in the United States, primarily in large cities, as well as throughout the world. The rise is mainly found in HIV-infected patients, in underrepresented ethnic groups, and in persons between the ages of 25 and 44. This risk to health is even more critical, since many of the infections involve mycobacteria that are resistant to some or all drugs that usually control TB.

Because infection is by exposure to contaminated aerosols, appropriate masks should be worn when one is exposed to a suspected coughing patient. Skin testing with PPD is suggested for health care workers to determine TB status, exposure, and seroconversion. Precautions and education are mandated by OSHA.

SUGGESTED READINGS

Necrotizing Ulcerative Gingivitis/Periodontitis

Lucatorto FM, Franker CK, Maza J: Postscaling Bacteremia in HIV-Associated Gingivitis and Periodontitis. Oral Surg Oral Med Oral Pathol 1992; 73:550-554.

Porter SR, Scully C, Luker J: Complications of Dental Surgery in Persons with HIV Disease. Oral Surg Oral Med Oral Pathol 1993; 75:165-167.

Rosenstein DI, Riviere GR, Elott KS: HIV-Associated Periodontal Disease: New Oral Spirochete Found. J Am Dent Assoc 1993; 124:76-80.

Winkler JR, Robertson PB: Periodontal Disease Associated with HIV Infection. Oral Surg Oral Med Oral Pathol 1992; 73:145-150.

Tuberculosis

Adal KA, Anglim AM, Palumbo CL, et al: The Use of High-Efficiency Particulate Air-Filter Respirators to Protect Hospital Workers from Tuberculosis: A Cost Effectiveness Analysis. N Engl J Med 1994; 331:169-173.

Centers for Disease Control: Tuberculosis Morbidity, United States, 1994. MMWR 1995; 44:387-395.

Shearer BG: MDR-TB: Another Challenge From the Microbial World. J Am Dent Assoc 1994; 12:43-49.

6   HIV-ASSOCIATED MALIGNANCIES

I t has been known for decades that immunocompromised persons are at risk for developing cancers. Therefore it is not surprising that HIV-infected individuals who have been immunodeficient for varying periods of time have an increased chance to develop malignancies. The most frequent is Kaposi's sarcoma, and non-Hodgkin's lymphomas show the fastest increasing prevalence. There also appears to be an increased risk to develop Hodgkin's lymphoma. Additionally, HIV-infected children are also at risk to develop malignancies.

KAPOSI'S SARCOMA (KS)

KS is a malignant reactive lesion, stemming from factors (cytokines) that induce the formation of tumors in widespread tissues and organs. The most prominent feature is produced by an angiogenesis factor, which in turn leads to the characteristic appearance of a vascular lesion.

While there has been a well-known endemic form of KS, occurring mainly in Africa and the northern Mediterranean area, epidemic KS associated with HIV immunodeficiency is much more lethal. Outside of immunosuppression, an exact etiology and all involved factors are unknown. Because KS is a reactive-type lesion, it is often considered a pseudomalignancy. KS can involve organs and be the cause of death, but most deaths in KS patients are due to opportunistic infections and the progressive wasting syndrome.

In the United States about 15% of all reported AIDS cases have KS as one of their AIDS-defining diseases. Although KS occurs in all AIDS groups, it is more frequent in homosexual and bisexual males, indicating special co-factors that may be preferentially transmitted by anal sex. The mean time of survival after the diagnosis of KS is about 2 years.

Diagnosis

Skin is the most common site of KS, but about half of patients will have oral KS. In many of these patients, oral KS may be the first or even the only manifestation. KS can afflict any oral mucosal site, with the palate being the most frequent and gingiva the second.

Initial manifestations appear as flat, red-purple, asymptomatic lesions. But since KS is a reactive response to cellular growth factors, the lesions increase in number and size, becoming nodular and symptomatic. KS can dramatically affect quality of life by esthetic blemishes, pain, bleeding, and interference with mouth functions.

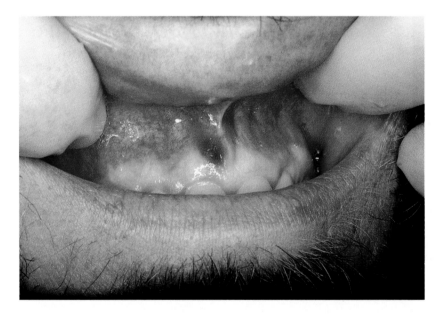

Figure 6.1 This 35-year-old, HIV-positive patient, who was otherwise without findings, developed an asymptomatic discolored spot on his anterior maxillary gingiva. The differential diagnosis included melanosis, hemangioma, injury, and purpura. A biopsy revealed Kaposi's sarcoma. This was the first sign of AIDS. A blood test showed his CD4 lymphocytes had dropped below 200 cells/μl, which is also an AIDS-defining condition.

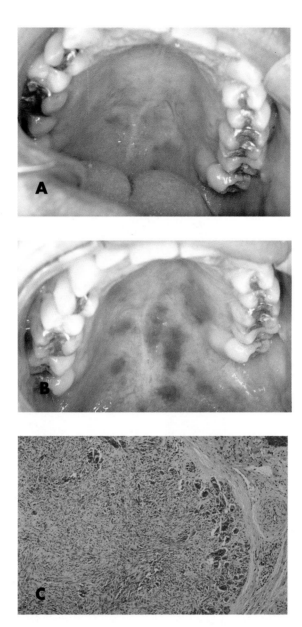

Figure 6.2 A, A 28-year-old HIV-positive male was seen because of a slight palatal irritation. He was otherwise asymptomatic. The very beginning signs of Kaposi's sarcoma were barely detectable. **B,** Two months later the lesions progressed to the characteristic features of KS. The flat, vascular-appearing palatal lesions reflected "growth factor" activity, stimulating lymphatic- and vascular-endothelial and fibroblastic proliferations. **C,** Biopsy of the palate confirmed KS and AIDS.

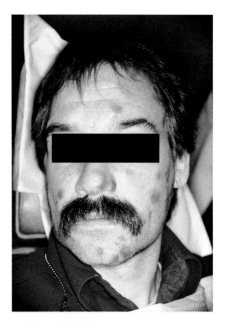

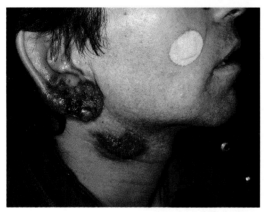

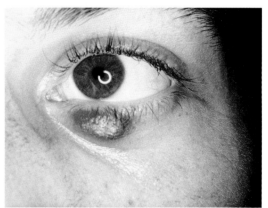

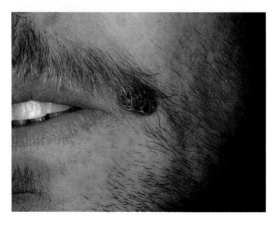

Figure 6.3 Kaposi's sarcoma of the skin in HIV-infected patients.

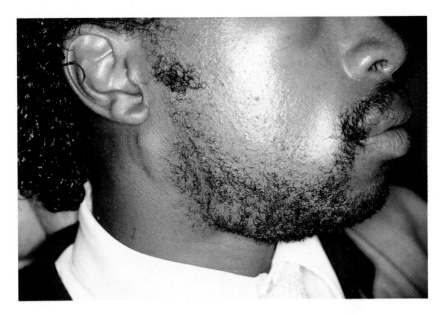

Figure 6.4 Kaposi's sarcoma involving a cervical lymph node.

Because of the variable clinical features, the differential diagnosis of KS can include hemangiomas, purpuric changes, and nonspecific inflammation. Bacillary angiomatosis can have a similar appearance, but this primarily cutaneous infection, caused by *Rochalimaea* bacteria, rarely occurs in oral mucosa. Diagnosis of KS is made by biopsy findings, which include connective tissue changes of vascular and fibrous proliferations and extravasation of red blood cells.

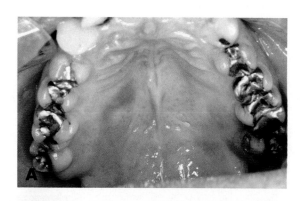

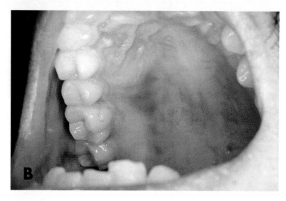

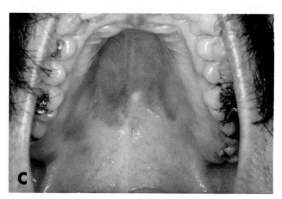

Figure 6.5 Various forms of Kaposi's sarcoma of the palate, which is the most common intraoral site. **A,** Very early, previously unnoticed, asymptomatic lesion of Kaposi's sarcoma. **B,** Slightly more extensive flat KS lesions, somewhat resembling ecchymosis of trauma, hemangioma, purpura, or even a minor salivary gland tumor. **C,** Extensive, flat KS, mildly symptomatic.

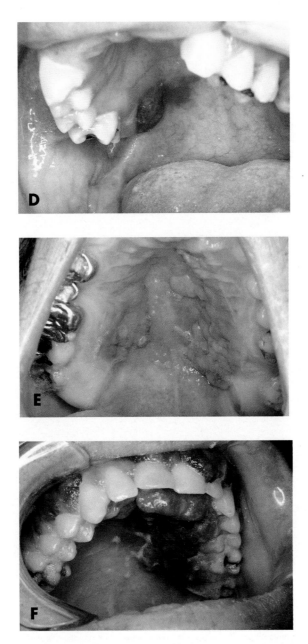

Figure 6.5—cont'd   D, Nodular KS. **E,** Widespread nodular KS. **F,** Advanced nodular KS, associated with pain and bleeding and interfering with speech and swallowing.

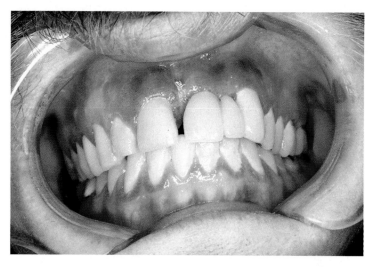

Figure 6.6 Flat, early Kaposi's sarcoma of upper gingiva. Note erythema of mandibular marginal gingiva, which is a non-KS gingivitis (linear marginal erythema).

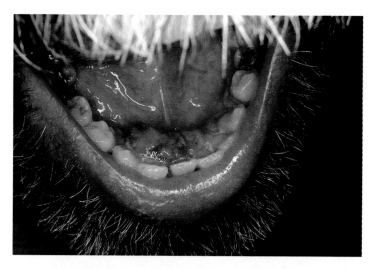

Figure 6.7 Nodular Kaposi's sarcoma involving the lower lingual gingiva.

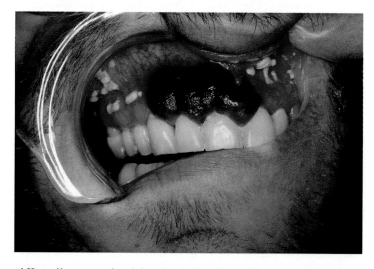

Figure 6.8 Advanced Kaposi's sarcoma involving the gingiva. Note adjacent candidal lesions.

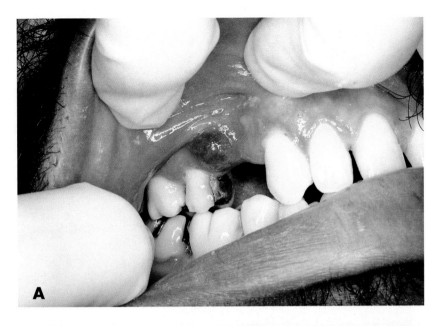

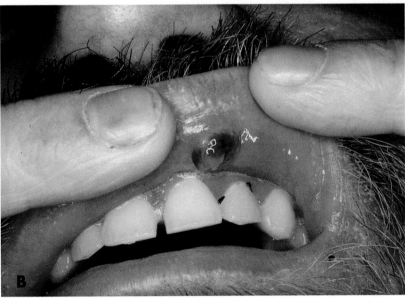

Figure 6.9 A, Kaposi's sarcoma of the gingiva resembling a hemangioma or blood-filled parulis. **B,** Kaposi's sarcoma of the labial mucosa resembling a hemangioma or a blood-filled pseudocyst.

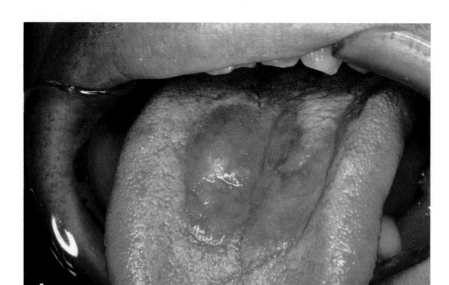

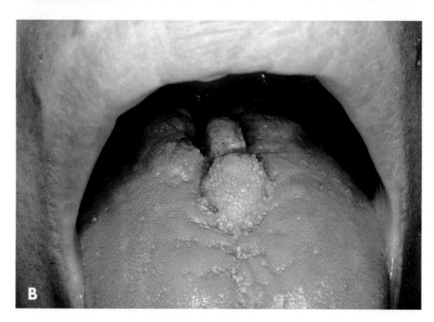

Figure 6.10 **A,** Kaposi's sarcoma involving the tongue. **B,** Kaposi's sarcoma occurring as "nonvascular"-appearing nodules.

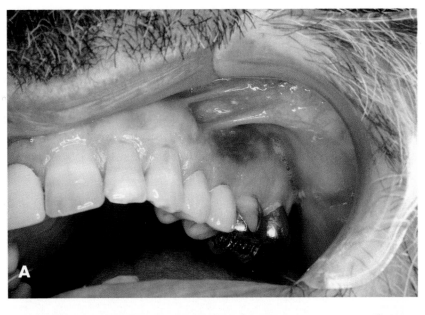

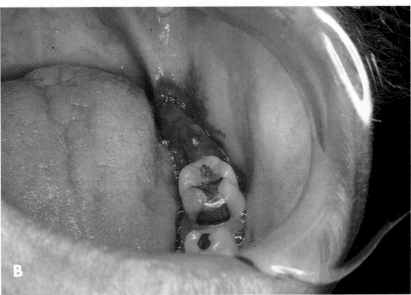

Figure 6.11 A, This Kaposi tumor was thought to be an atypical amalgam deposition or melanosis by the referring clinician. **B,** This Kaposi tumor was mistaken for a hemangioma.

Treatment

When lesions are widespread, systemic chemotherapy is helpful. For oral lesion that are well localized, intralesional injections (the cytotoxic drug, vinblastine, or the sclerosing agent, sodium tetradecyl sulfate) are effective. Surgery is possible but not recommended. For more extensive oral involvement, low-dose radiation has been useful (total dosages usually do not exceed 1500 cGy). In any case, treatment objectives are to reduce signs and symptoms and are almost never curative. Again, the choice of treatment depends on patient desires, cost, time, and other criteria for compliance. While treatment of oral KS can improve quality of life, there is no indication that it alters survival.

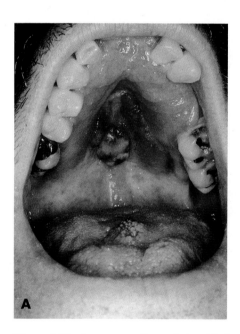

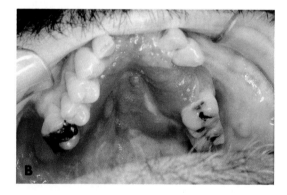

Figure 6.12 An accurate diagnosis is critical, since hemangiomas, mucosal trauma, purpuric lesions, and infections can resemble Kaposi's sarcoma (KS). **A,** This painful vascular-appearing lesion in an HIV-positive patient resembled KS. It had been noticed for 2 weeks and would have signaled the terminal phase of HIV infection. A biopsy was only suggestive of KS. **B,** Because of an acute dental infection, the patient was given 2 g pencillin V daily for 1 week, which led to remission in signs and symptoms. The retrospective diagnosis was that of bacillary angiomatosis.

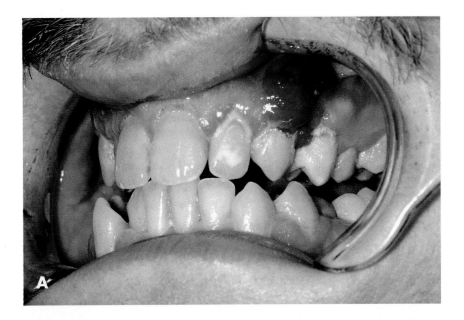

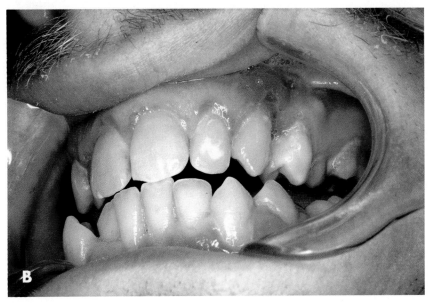

Figure 6.13 A, A painful, hemorrhagic, nodular Kaposi's sarcoma of the gingiva that was increasing in size. **B,** Two weeks after one radiation treatment of 800 cGy the tumor was flat and asymptomatic. Although not cured, the lesion remained unchanged for the remaining 8 months that the patient lived.

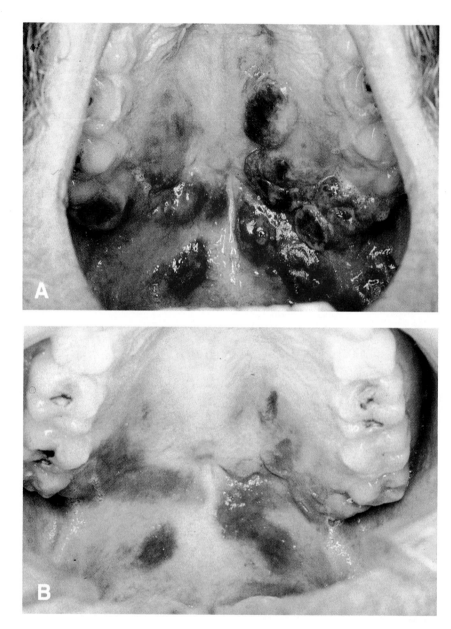

Figure 6.14 A, Painful extensive Kaposi's sarcoma of the palate and oropharynx. **B,** Remission of signs and symptoms following radiation therapy (1500 cGy in 10 days).

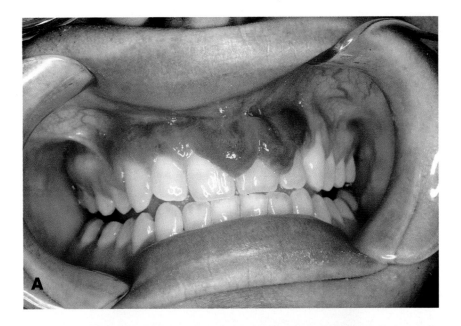

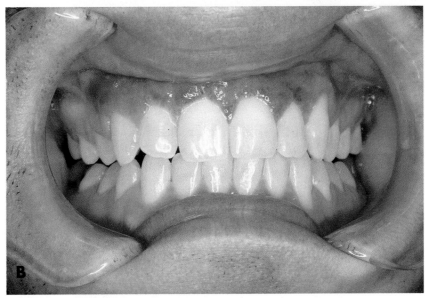

Figure 6.15 A, Painful and esthetically undesirable Kaposi's sarcoma of the gingiva. **B,** Three weeks following removal by CO_2 laser.

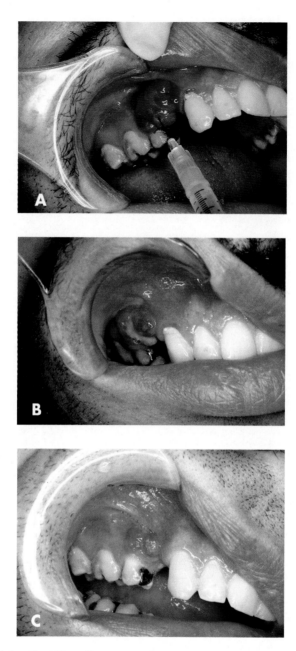

Figure 6.16 A, A painful, localized Kaposi's sarcoma of the gingiva that was enlarging and becoming hemorrhagic. The patient's CD4 count was 130. Local injections of a sclerosing agent (3% sodium tetradecyl sulfate) were administered by multiple "sticks." **B,** One week later the tumor had ulcerated and remained painful. **C,** Two weeks later, the lesion became asymptomatic and had dramatically decreased in size. There was no regrowth after a 3-month follow-up.

NON-HODGKIN'S LYMPHOMA (NHL)

As expected, the occurrence of NHL continues to increase as the number of HIV-infected people grows and their longevity extends. Inappropriate B-lymphocyte stimulation and the presence of Epstein-Barr virus play a role, but all the co-factors are poorly understood.

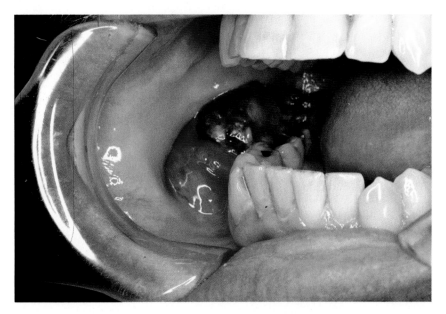

Figure 6.17 This 25-year-old gay male was seen for facial swelling and a rapidly growing gingivobuccal mass. The patient had noticed the problem for "less than 2 months." He denied any past history of diseases or the use of any drugs. Biopsy proved the lesion to be a non-Hodgkin's lymphoma, which prompted HIV serology with resultant positive findings.

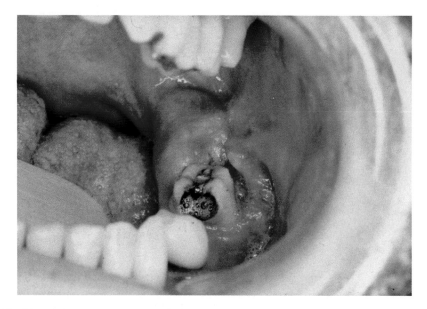

Figure 6.18 This painful swelling in the mandibular retromolar area was thought to be due to a dental abscess in the 30-year-old homosexual nurse. When there was no response to antibiotics, a biopsy was obtained that revealed non-Hodgkin's lymphoma. The patient died from disseminated disease 4 months later. He was HIV-positive.

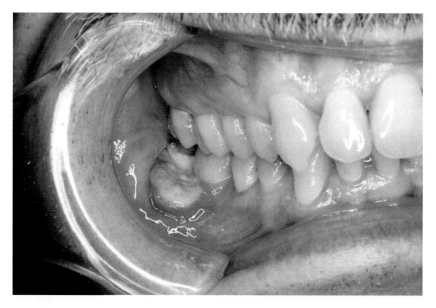

Figure 6.19 This 62-year-old patient became HIV-infected from a blood transfusion during heart surgery 8 years before. He was asymptomatic until 1 month prior to this visit, when he noticed some unintentional weight loss and a gingival "infection." Based on a negative dental x-ray and no response to an antibiotic, a biopsy was performed. The diagnosis was non-Hodgkin's lymphoma. This was the first sign of disseminated lymphoma and a markedly declining CD4 count. He died 2 months after aggressive radiation and chemotherapy.

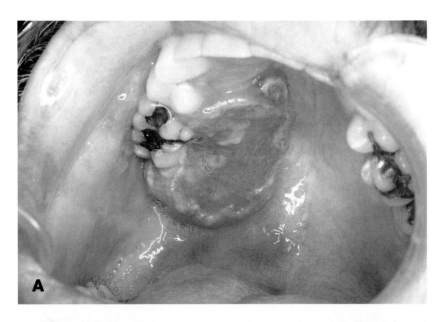

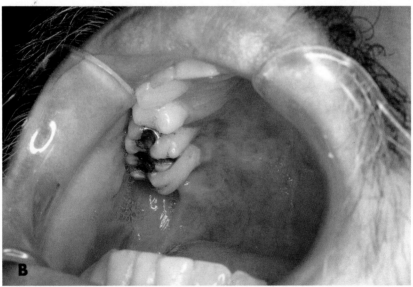

Figure 6.20 A, This 38-year-old HIV-infected patient was referred because of a painful gingivopalatal ulceration that had doubled in size in less than 2 weeks. He was otherwise asymptomatic. A biopsy showed non-Hodgkin's lymphoma. **B,** An aggressive 12-week course of multicytotoxic drugs led to remission. The patient survived less than 1 year.

Frequently these lymphomas are extranodal and can involve the mouth. In some cases, oral NHL has been either the first or the only evidence of NHL tumor. Oral NHL can appear as masses or ulcerative lesions. This diversity of appearance again mandates an imaginative differential diagnosis, so that significant lesions will be properly diagnosed and managed. Biopsy is necessary for a definitive diagnosis, classification, staging, and treatment. While KS is a more common malignancy in gay men, NHL is more common in HIV heterosexual drug users.

Treatment must be aggressive for optimal results. Two-year survival rates are poor, approximating 20%. Multiple cytotoxic drugs offer the best results. This added immunosuppression obviously increases the complications during and after therapy. These complications include other oral diseases, such as thrush, aphthous-like lesions, and lichenoid reactions.

SQUAMOUS CARCINOMA

Oral squamous carcinoma usually occurs beyond the fourth decade in life, with the mean age being about 62. However, in the HIV patient, squamous carcinomas have been diagnosed not too infrequently, and the mean age has been in the third decade of life. These occurrences indicate that oral squamous carcinoma is probably an HIV-associated malignancy. The characteristics have been rapid growth and poor therapeutic responses to both radiation and surgery.

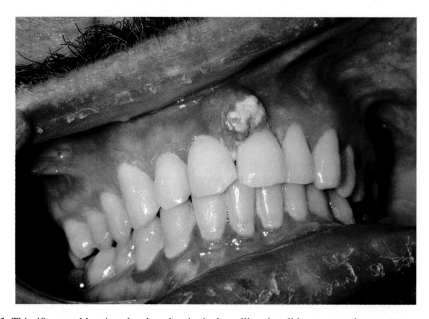

Figure 6.21 This 40-year-old patient developed a gingival swelling that did not respond to curettage, mouth rinses, and antibiotics. A biopsy revealed squamous carcinoma. The tumor was treated with radiation.

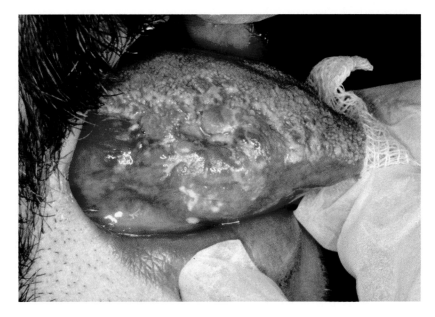

Figure 6.22 Squamous carcinoma of the tongue in a 30-year-old homosexual man. He also was a moderately heavy smoker and drinker. Two years later he was shown to be HIV-infected. Note also pseudomembranous candidiasis.

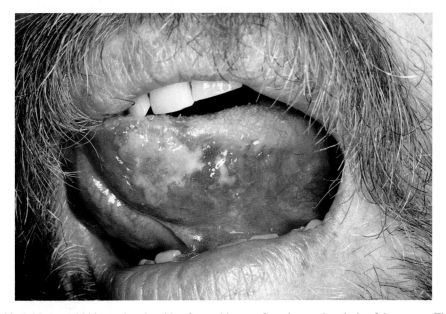

Figure 6.23 A 32-year-old bisexual male with a 2-year history of erosive erythroplasia of the tongue. The anterior portion of the lesion revealed squamous carcinoma. The patient also had a history of venereal disease, hepatitis, and marijuana abuse.

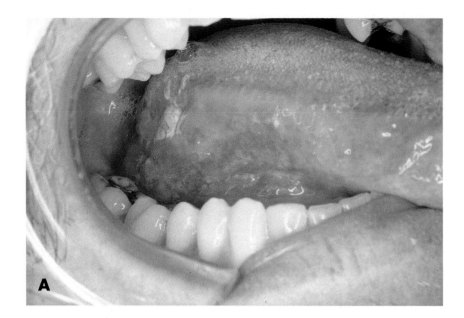

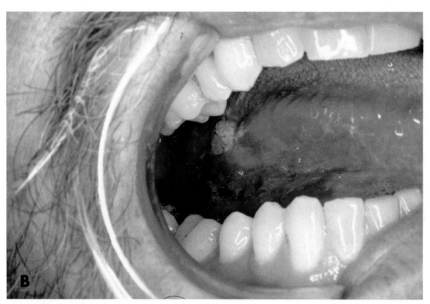

Figure 6.24 A, A 26-year-old HIV-positive homosexual man sought consultation because of a mild irritation of the right posterior tongue. A moderately firm erythroplastic lesion was noted inferior to an area of leukoplakia. His history was positive for venereal disease, hepatitis, and candidiasis. **B,** The erythematous portion of the lesion retained stain after an application of 1% toluidine blue dye and resisted decolorization with 1% acetic acid. A biopsy from the erythroplasia revealed squamous carcinoma. A combination of surgery and radiation did not control the carcinoma, and he died 1 year later.

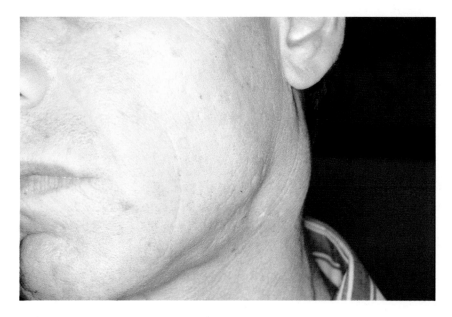

Figure 6.25 This 36-year-old, HIV-positive patient noticed a lump in his neck that was progressively increasing in size and discomfort over a 2-month period. The differential diagnosis included dental infection, lymphoepithelial cyst, parotid gland lesion, and tumor. A fine needle aspiration biopsy showed this to be a squamous carcinoma involving a lymph node, with the primary carcinoma arising in the hypopharynx.

These carcinomas seem to arise de novo without evidence of premalignant changes, such as leukoplakia or erythroplakia. While the tongue appears to be the most common intraoral site, there has been no association with oral hairy leukoplakia. However, co-factors seem to include histories of smoking and alcohol habits. Viral influence on proto-oncogenes, growth factors, and suppressor proteins has not been established.

SUGGESTED READING

Kaposi's Sarcoma

Epstein J, Silverman S Jr: HIV-Associated Malignancies. Oral Surg Oral Med Oral Pathol 1992; 73:193-200.

Lucatorto FM, Sapp JP: Treatment of Oral Kaposi's Sarcoma with a Sclerosing Agent in AIDS Patients. Oral Surg Oral Med Oral Pathol 1993; 75:192-198.

Moore PS, Chang Y: Detection of Herpesvirus-Like DNA Sequences in Kaposi's Sarcoma in Patients with and Those without HIV Infection. N Engl J Med 1995; 332:1181-1185.

Nichols CM, Flaitz CM, Hicks MJ: Treating Kaposi's Lesions in the HIV-Infected Patient. J Am Dent Assoc 1993; 124:78- 84.

Regezi JA, MacPhail LA, Daniels TE, et al: Oral Kaposi's Sarcoma: a 10-Year Retrospective Histopathologic Study. J Oral Pathol Med 1993; 22:292-297.

Non-Hodgkin's Lymphoma

Arico M, Caselli D, D'Argenio P, et al: Malignancies in Children with Human Immunodeficiency Virus Type 1 Infection. Cancer 1991; 68:2473-2477.

Armitage JO: Treatment of Non-Hodgkin's Lymphoma. N Engl J Med 1993; 328:1023-1030.

Hicks MJ, Flaitz CM, Nichols CM, et al: Intraoral Presentation of Anaplastic Large-Cell Ki-1 Lymphoma in Association with HIV Infection. Oral Surg Oral Med Oral Pathol 1993; 76:73-81.

Rubio R: Hodgkin's Disease Associated with Human Immunodeficiency Virus Infection: A Clinical Study of 46 Cases. Cancer 1994; 73:2400-2407.

Safai B, Diaz B, Schwartz J: Malignant Neoplasms Associated with Human Immunodeficiency Virus Infection. CA 1992; 42:74-95.

7

OTHER HIV-ASSOCIATED LESIONS

HIV immunodeficiency has complicated the differential diagnosis of oral lesions because of the multitude of diverse signs and symptoms associated with known oral diseases that in the immunocompromised can occur with more severe forms, as well as new oral conditions that are not clearly classified. This complicates management, since optimal treatment depends on an accurate diagnosis. In turn, a successful outcome also depends on knowledge of therapeutic approaches and host factors, which include status of immune competence/staging, other current diseases/conditions being treated, and capability for patient compliance regarding the treatment plan.

RECURRENT APHTHOUS-LIKE STOMATITIS

All present data indicate that recurrent aphthous ulcerations (RAS) are a reflection of an autoimmune abnormality. In the general population, where occurrence varies between 20% and 40%, there seems to be a genetic influence. In any case, and in all probability, molecules formed on the surface of some epithelial cells attract lymphocytes that in turn lead to the manifestations of RAS. Based on these findings, and in the absence of any other evident causative factors, RAS is classified as an immunologic disorder.

In the HIV patient, RAS attacks can occur for the first time without any previous history; in those who have an RAS history, the lesions can occur more frequently and in more severe forms. The increased severity includes multiple ulcerations and/or larger lesions (major aphthae). The more severe RAS are referred to as aphthous-like, since the diverse appearances can be mistaken for cancers, granulomatous diseases, or a variety of infections. Obviously, this complicates the diagnosis, which in turn often delays the correct therapeutic management through the use of ineffective medications. Therefore, in many cases, the diagnosis is finally reached by ruling out other conditions. Because of the frequently seen unusual appearances, biopsy may be the first diagnostic choice.

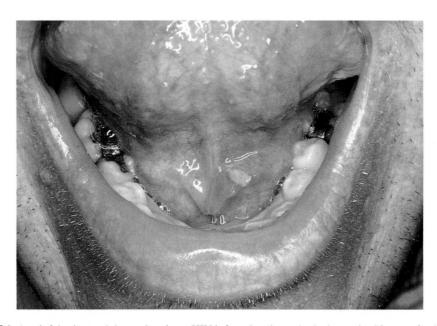

Figure 7.1 A painful minor aphthous ulcer in an HIV-infected patient who had no prior history of aphthae.

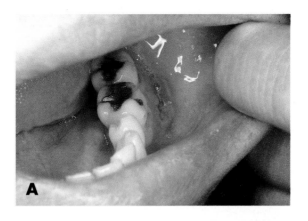

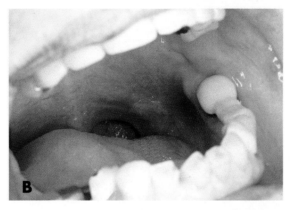

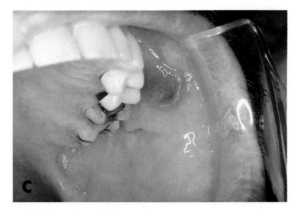

Figure 7.2 Major aphthae in otherwise asymptomatic HIV-positive patients. These large aphthae persist for months, are very painful, and usually require anti-inflammatory corticosteroid treatment for effective control. **A,** Buccal-gingival reflex. **B,** Mandibular retromolar gingiva. **C,** Buccal mucosa.

continued

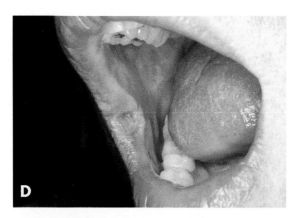

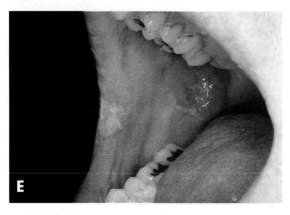

Figure 7.2—cont'd This AIDS patient has started to develop more frequent and severe recurrent aphthous-like ulcers. **D,** An ulcer on his right commissure persisted for 2 weeks without any evidence of healing. A decrease in signs and symptoms followed 5 days of prednisone (80 mg daily). **E,** A few days following the prednisone treatment, he developed another acutely painful ulcer on his right buccal mucosa. A biopsy was consistent with a benign ulceration, and the lesion responded to 80 mg of daily prednisone after 7 days. His immune deficiency was accelerating, and he died from *Pneumocystis carinii* pneumonia 4 months later.

Treatment is often mandatory based on the degree of pain, which may be almost intolerable and preclude adequate nutritional intake. This can lead to acute weight loss, malaise, depression, and increased susceptibility to infections. The most effective treatment is use of corticosteroids to alter the T-lymphocytes attracted to the site that are critical participants in the immunologic reaction. Adverse side effects should be understood and discussed with patients, and the primary care physicians should concur with the treatment regimen.

Systemic corticosteroids are more predictable and prompt better patient compliance. Our studies have shown that high-dose, short course use usually leads to beneficial results within a week without any clinical or laboratory evidence of aggravating immune incompetence, no matter what the level of CD4 cells might be. Therefore, daily dosages of prednisone vary between 40 and 80 mg. When used less than 10 to 14 days, the dosage is never tapered. Duration of therapy depends on control of signs and symptoms.

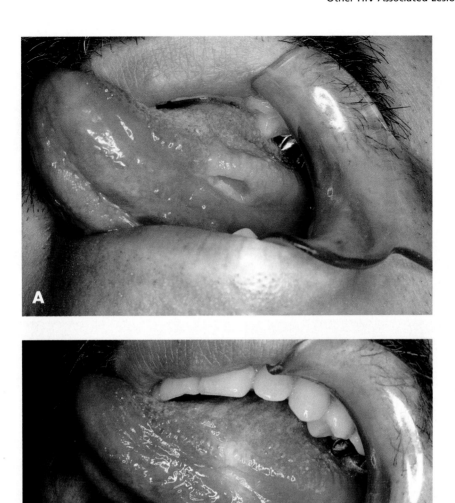

Figure 7.3 A, This 37-year-old HIV-infected homosexual presented with an indurated, painful ulcer of 3 weeks duration. A biopsy was considered to rule out tumor or a granulomatous disease. However, because of a past history of aphthae, he was started on a trial of prednisone, 60 mg daily. **B,** At 6 days the ulcer had healed and he was asymptomatic, so the prednisone was discontinued.

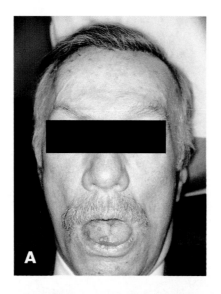

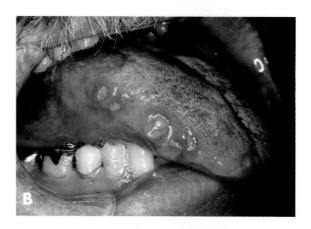

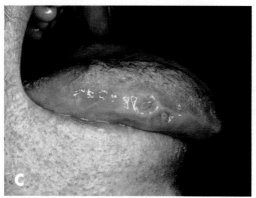

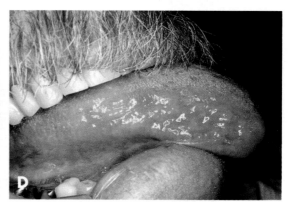

Figure 7.4 A and **B,** This 41-year-old bisexual was referred because of persistent, painful tongue ulcers present for almost 3 weeks. The pain prevented normal dietary intake and 15 pounds were unintentionally lost. He had no other current complaints and was not taking any medications except morphine for the pain. He was started on 60 mg prednisone daily. **C,** In 4 days he had a dramatic resolution of the ulcers and very little discomfort. His food intake returned to normal. **D,** At 7 days there was complete healing. However, this attack signaled a decline in his CD4 function and count, and he soon developed opportunistic infections and died 6 months later. The correct classification was Behcet's syndrome, since the patient had mild arthritis and ulcers on his penis that healed while he was taking the prednisone.

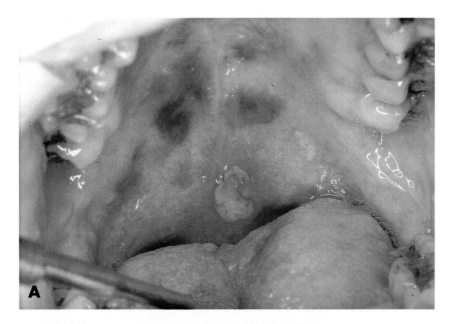

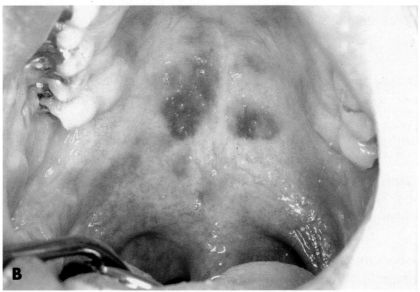

Figure 7.5 A, This AIDS patient had Kaposi's sarcoma of the palate along with a major aphthous ulcer of soft palate, persisting for 2 weeks and "getting worse." Because of the pain, he was not eating and already had lost 12 pounds, which was further compromising his prognosis. He was stable prior to the ulcer. After 3 days of 60 mg prednisone daily, the symptoms were minimal and the patient was again eating. **B,** After 1 week of treatment, the lesion had completely healed.

As an alternative, topical corticosteroids can be utilized either therapeutically or prophylactically. However, because of the difficulty in maintaining sufficient contact time, the more potent corticosteroids must be utilized. These would include fluocinonide (0.05%, Lidex) and clobetosol (0.05%, Temovate). They can be mixed with equal parts of Orabase for adherence. Fluocinonide also comes as a 0.05% gel, which some patients prefer. Corticosteroids in the form of mouth rinses are sometimes helpful, for example, elixir of Decadron (dexamethasone, 0.5 mg/5 ml) 1 tablespoon held in the mouth for 1 to 2 minutes, then emptied, about 3 times daily.

Studies have indicated that corticosteroids markedly alter cytokine production of lymphocytes, which in turn diminishes the response and allows epithelial healing and elimination of pain. Sometimes antifungal medications must be used prophylactically because corticosteroids promote conversion of glycogen to glucose, which fosters fungal growth by adding substrate for proliferation.

Other modulators of T-lymphocyte function, such as cyclosporine, thalidomide, and levamisole, are not practical for one or more reasons including cost, inadequate clinical studies, toxicity, hypersensitivity, and availability.

HYPERSENSITIVITY AND LICHENOID REACTION

Stemming from the decreased cell-mediated and humoral immunity, acquired allergies are commonly found in advanced HIV immune dysregulation. The reactions can be based on autoimmune reactions or adverse responses to drugs, food, or environmental factors.

The diagnosis is based on history and clinical findings. The lesions may appear similar to erythema multiforme (erythematous, irregular ulcerations covered by pseudomembranes, painful) or to lichen planus (keratotic striations, erythema, ulcerations, bothersome to painful). When allergic-type reactions are suspected, a trial of corticosteroids will help confirm the diagnosis as well as initiate treatment. As stated previously for RAS, systemic corticosteroids are more predictable, but topicals can be used as an alternative. If this approach is used, and in the absence of a satisfactory response, further diagnostic approaches must be used to establish a diagnosis. Biopsy is helpful in confirming and/or ruling out various other entities.

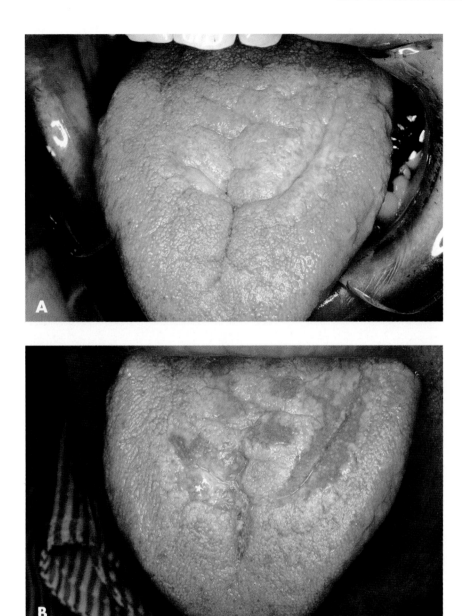

Figure 7.6 This 36-year-old homosexual man who had been HIV-infected for 2 years developed oral discomfort. The tongue lesion was biopsied and found to be clinically and histologically consistent with lichen planus. Culture of the mouth and special staining of the biopsy specimen revealed no evidence of *Candida*. **B,** The lesion has persisted for more than 1 year and periodically becomes erythematous (atrophic form of lichen planus). Short 2- to 3-day courses of prednisone (40 mg/day) would control the signs and symptoms.

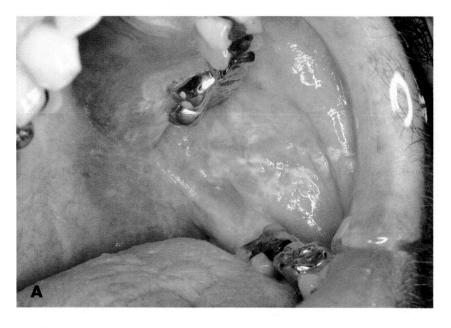

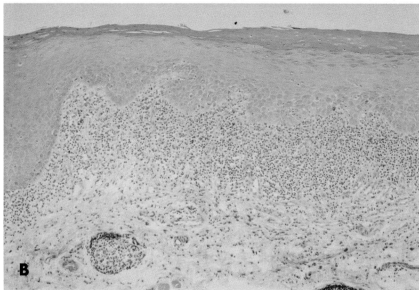

Figure 7.7 A, This AIDS patient with Kaposi's sarcoma of the palate developed asymptomatic reticular keratoses of the buccal mucosa and palate. There was no evident causative factor. **B,** A biopsy revealed a lichenoid-type reaction.

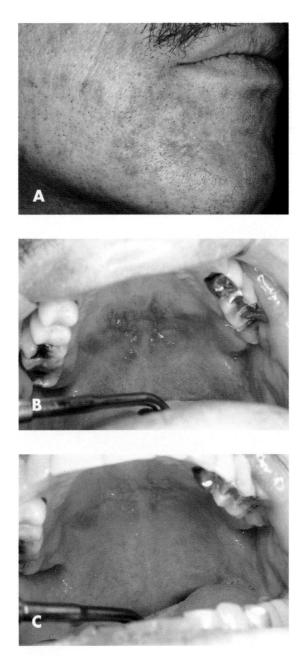

Figure 7.8 This 33-year-old HIV-positive heterosexual was referred because of palatal pain lasting 1 week. He had no other complaints and his CD4 count had been stable around 300. Examination revealed a concomitant skin rash (**A**) and a diffuse palatal erythema (**B**). **C,** After 5 days of 40 mg prednisone daily, the oral and skin signs/symptoms disappeared. The impression was idiopathic erythema multiforme. There were no adverse side effects from the treatment, which was discontinued after day 5. Subsequent recurrences responded similarly.

SIALADENITIS AND XEROSTOMIA

Xerostomia, reflecting a complaint of dryness that is usually associated with salivary gland hypofunction, is a not uncommon complaint in HIV-infected patients. This may or may not be coincidental with salivary gland enlargement. The most common glands involved are the parotids. The major significance is related to the promotion of candidiasis by a xerostomic environment, which also reflects in all probability a corresponding diminution of antifungal salivary proteins.

The cause of either glandular enlargement and/or salivary hypofunction is not known. However, based on the predisposition to autoimmune disease, lymphocytic infiltration of the salivary glands may suppress the cells that produce saliva, thus rendering a Sjogren's-like syndrome. Alternatively, cytomegalovirus presence and infections are common in HIV patients. Since this virus has a predilection for salivary gland tissue, the xerostomia may be the indirect reflection of a viral infection, with the basic factor being one of immunosuppression.

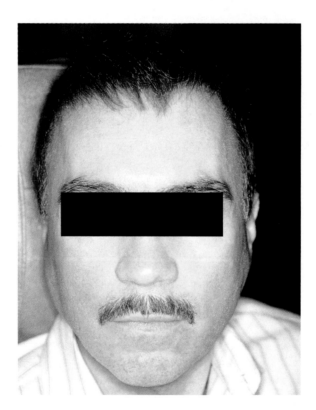

Figure 7.9 This HIV-infected patient had mildly symptomatic, chronic, bilateral parotid gland swelling for more than 2 years. Cultures were negative for any infectious microbial organism and a fine needle aspiration biopsy was negative for lymphoma. Causative factors and long-term prognosis are unknown. Treatment is symptomatic. This might represent an autoimmune inflammatory salivary gland response or a response to the presence of cytomegalovirus.

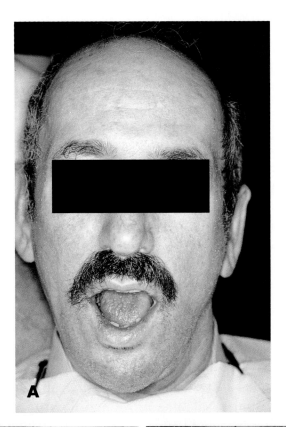

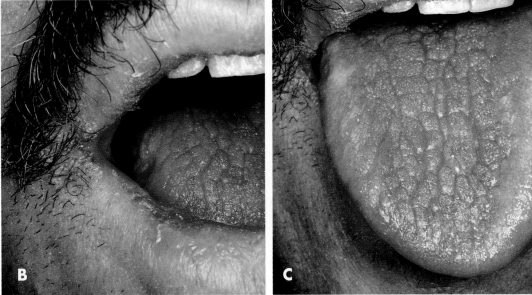

Figure 7.10 A, This healthy appearing business executive was referred because of a dry mouth. His recorded health history was unremarkable and he used no drugs. Examination revealed angular cheilitis **(B)**, observable xerostomia, and a fissured tongue **(C)**. Because of the sudden onset, immunosuppression was considered, leading to serology and a positive HIV result. The signs and symptoms were improved by daily pilocarpine to increase saliva and antifungals for the associated candidiasis.

The diagnosis is established on the basis of clinical findings and ruling out other diseases. Considerations include infection, inflammation, tumor, and lymphoepithelial cysts. Infection can be ruled out by the use of antibiotics and neoplasia utilizing fine needle aspiration biopsy. The most frequent finding is that of benign idiopathic hyperplasia.

There is no definitive or reproducibly effective treatment. Therefore, the approach is symptomatic management. This involves keeping the mouth as moist as possible and maintaining optimal hygiene. The simplest approach is the use of frequent water rinses, antiseptic mouth rinses, and sugarless gum or candy. Physiologic saliva stimulation can be attained by the sialogogues, pilocarpine (Salagen, 5 mg three to four times daily) or bethanechol (Urecholine, 25 to 50 mg three to four times daily).

THROMBOCYTOPENIA

Many HIV-positive patients produce inappropriate antibodies directed against their own platelets. This thrombocytopenia can lead to easily induced or even spontaneous submucosal bleeding, leading to purpuric discoloration (thrombocytopenia purpura) and hematomas. Therefore, the lowered number of blood platelets can cause some problems with hemostasis and swelling following invasive or traumatic dental procedures.

The first line of treatment is the use of corticosteroids. If this approach is unsuccessful, then splenectomy is considered.

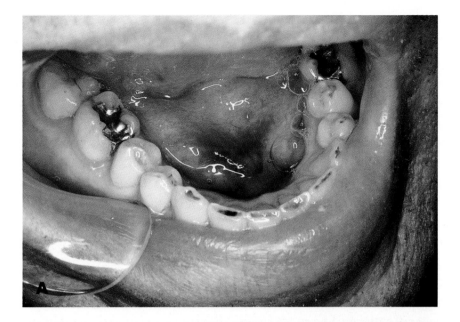

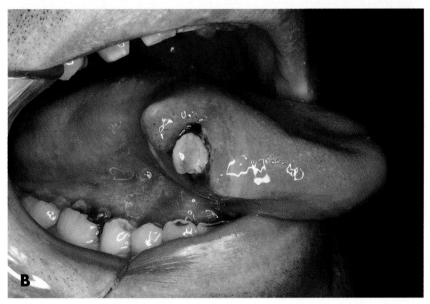

Figure 7.11 A, This HIV-positive drug abuser had generalized toxoplasmosis with central nervous system involvement. His platelet count was less than 50,000/mm^3. Note the purpuric lesion in the floor of his mouth (thrombocytopenic purpura). **B,** During a seizure he bit his tongue, inducing a necrotic ulcer and hematoma.

ULCERATIVE STOMATITIS AND UNCLASSIFIED LESIONS

Occasionally HIV patients present with ulcerations that are frequently necrotic, progressive, and painful. In spite of biopsies and cultures, definitive diagnoses remain uncertain. While there might well be associated secondary infection, antibiotics alone are not curative. Since corticosteroids are not helpful, there is no basis to classify such lesions as atypical aphthae. Because these ulcerations usually occur in advanced immunodeficiency, they may simply be due to idiopathic tissue necrosis or even advanced programmed cell death (apoptosis).

Management approaches include ruling out a definitive diagnosis, palliation and general supportive care, empirical trials with medications, consideration of debridement, and follow-up.

Infrequently, other mucosal changes occur that do not fit any established disease classifications. The most practical approach is to rule out known disease entities, treat symptoms (if any) empirically, and follow the patient.

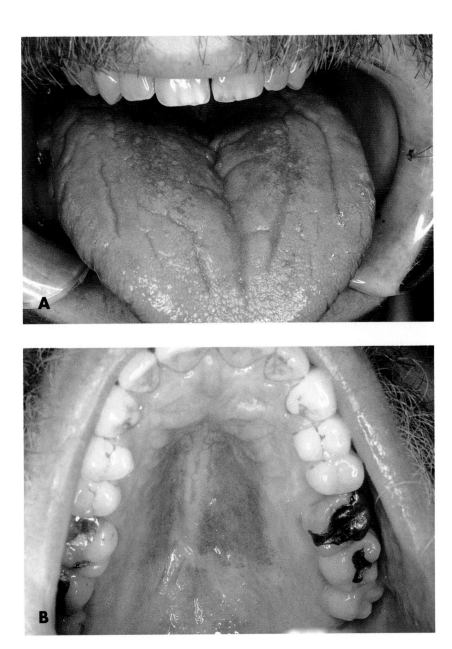

Figure 7.12 These telangiectatic lesions on the dorsal tongue **(A)** and palate **(B)** were asymptomatic and chronic; they were present consistently for more than 1 year without change in this AIDS patient. A biopsy showed a nonspecific mucositis and all other tests were noncontributory. Also, there was no correlation between medical status or habits. The significance of these not-too-infrequent mucosal changes is unknown.

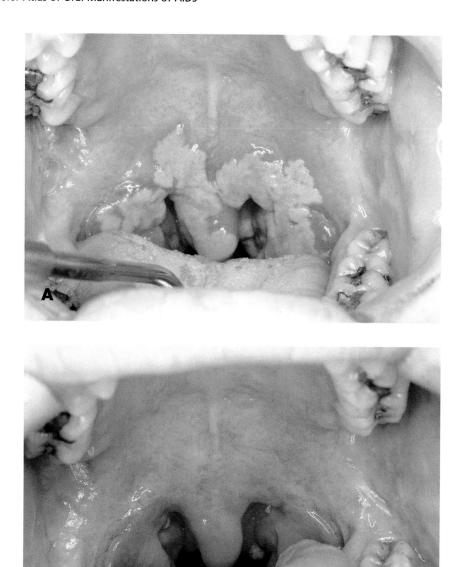

Figure 7.13 A, This oropharyngeal pseudomembranous lesion was present without change in this 26-year-old HIV-positive patient for 4 months. Cultures were negative for virus, *Candida,* or predominant bacterial pathogens. A biopsy revealed a nonspecific mucositis. No treatment was instituted because the lesion did not bother the patient. **B,** All signs spontaneously disappeared during the fifth month.

Oral hyperpigmentation (melanotic macules), appearing in a variety of configurations, have been associated with HIV infection. However, the occurrence has not been significantly greater than developing melanotic macules in control groups. The importance remains an enigma. These depositions of pigment and/or melanin may be responses to various medications or alterations in adrenal steroids.

There have been isolated reports of a variety of oral conditions possibly related to HIV immunodeficiency. But until well-designed and controlled studies are carried out, a definitive association rather than a coincidental relationship remains speculative.

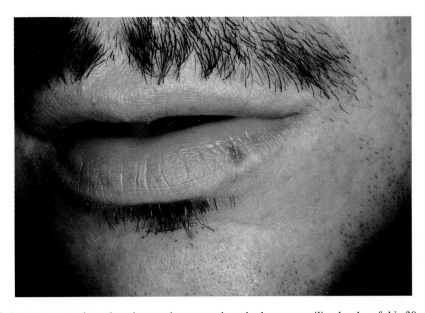

Figure 7.14 An asymptomatic melanotic macule appeared on the lower vermilion border of this 30-year-old gay man. The association, if any, with HIV infection is not known and not related to the CD4 count or any specific disease entity.

NUTRITIONAL CONSIDERATIONS

Unintentional weight loss of more than 10% (wasting syndrome) is an AIDS-defining disease, a sign of declining immunocompetency, and a leading cause of death. Therefore, good nutrition to maintain weight is critically important. Optimal oral health to obviate infection and pain becomes a substantial factor in dietary intake. Urging a high-caloric consumption in addition to maintaining an appetite will contribute to both quality and length of survival. However, the basic cause is related to poorly understood factors involving both gastrointestinal absorption of nutrients and metabolism.

SUGGESTED READINGS

Recurrent Aphthous Stomatitis

MacPhail LA, Greenspan D, Greenspan JS: Recurrent Aphthous Ulcers in Association with HIV Infection: Diagnosis and Treatment. Oral Surg Oral Med Oral Pathol 1992; 73:283-288.

Muzyka BC, Glick M: Major Aphthous Ulcers in Patients with HIV Disease. Oral Surg Oral Med Oral Pathol 1994; 77:116-120.

Silverman S Jr, Gallo J, Stites DP: Prednisone Management of HIV-Associated Recurrent Oral Aphthous Ulcerations. J Acquir Immun Defic Syndr 1992; 5:952-953.

Hypersensitivity and Lichenoid Reactions

Bayard PJ, Berger TG, Jacobson MA: Drug Hypersensitivity Reactions and Human Immunodeficiency Virus Disease. J Acquir Immun Defic Syndr 1992; 5:1237-1257.

Coopman SA, Johnson RA, Platt R, Stern RS: Cutaneous Disease and Drug Reactions in HIV Infection. N Engl J Med 1993; 328:1670-1674.

Ficarra G, Flaitz CM, Gaglioti D, et al: White Lichenoid Lesions of the Buccal Mucosa in Patients with HIV Infection. Oral Surg Oral Med Oral Pathol 1993; 76:460-466.

Grinspoon SK, Bilezikian JP: HIV Disease and the Endocrine System. N Engl J Med 1992; 327:1360-1365.

Kumar M, Kumar AM, Morgan R, et al: Abnormal Pituitary- Adrenocortical Response in Early HIV-1 Infection. J Acquir Immun Defic Syndr 1993; 6:61-65.

Sialadenitis and Xerostomia

Muller F, Holberg-Petersen M, Rollag H, et al: Nonspecific Oral Immunity in Individuals with HIV Infection. J Acquir Immun Defic Syndr 1992; 5:46-51.
Pollock JJ, Santarpia RP III, Heller HM, et al: Determination of Salivary Anticandidal Activities in Healthy Adults and Patients with AIDS: A Pilot Study. J Acquir Immun Defic Syndr 1992; 5:610-618.
Schiodt M, Dodd CL, Greenspan D, et al: Natural History of HIV-Associated Salivary Gland Disease. Oral Surg Oral Med Oral Pathol 1992; 74:326-331.

Thrombocytopenia

Rigaud M, Leibovitz E, Quee CS, et al: Thrombocytopenia in Children Infected with Human Immunodeficiency Virus: Long-Term Follow-Up and Therapeutic Considerations. J Acquir Immun Defic Syndr 1992; 5:450-455.

Nutrition

Abrams B, Duncan D, Hertz-Picciotto I: A Prospective Study of Dietary Intake and Acquired Immune Deficiency Syndrome in HIV-Seropositive Homosexual Men. J Acquir Immun Defic Syndr 1993; 6:949-958.
Graham KK, Mikolich DJ, Fisher AE, et al: Pharmacologic Evaluation of Megestrol Acetate Oral Suspension in Cachectic AIDS Patients. J Acquir Immun Defic Syndr 1994; 7:580-586.
Slusarczyk R: The Influence of the Human Immunodeficiency Virus on Resting Energy Expenditure. J Acquir Immun Defic Syndr 1994; 7:1025-1027.

8

CASE PRESENTATIONS

$\mathbf{A}$s already discussed and illustrated, progressive HIV immunodeficiency fosters patient susceptibility to opportunistic infections, immunologic diseases/conditions, and malignancies. The oral cavity has a significant role, since the first signs and symptoms of HIV infection may occur in the mouth. Often these oral manifestations become chief complaints for varying periods of time, and not too infrequently they signal an accelerated decline of immune competence and advanced AIDS.

Therefore the health care provider becomes involved in a diverse spectrum of diagnoses, treatments, consultations, and referrals. A general knowledge of most aspects of HIV infection, an understanding of pathogenesis and progression, information regarding referral facilities, and compassion for mental as well as physical status are all essential to satisfactorily caring for HIV patients and practicing optimal standards of care.

The purpose of this chapter is to illustrate many of the diverse clinical features of HIV infection and progression of disease. These examples will demonstrate some of the various roles that health care workers can provide in caring for HIV-infected patients.

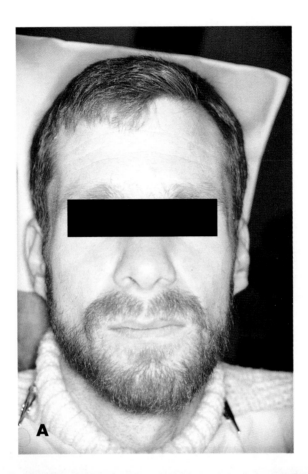

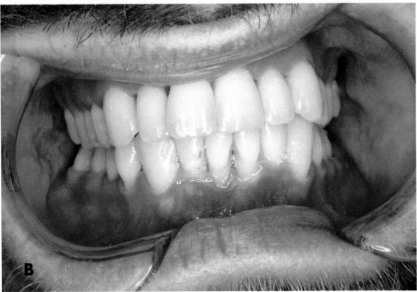

Figure 8.1 A, This apparently healthy 27-year-old man reported to the clinic with a chief complaint of mildly sore gums. Medical history included hepatitis B, venereal infections, and sporadic use of cocaine, marijuana, amyl nitrate, and alcohol. He had experienced no previous weight loss, malaise, or night sweats. **B,** Findings included gingival recession and alveolar bone loss involving teeth #24 and #25 in particular and blunted-ulcerated interdental papillae. Hygiene was good.

continued

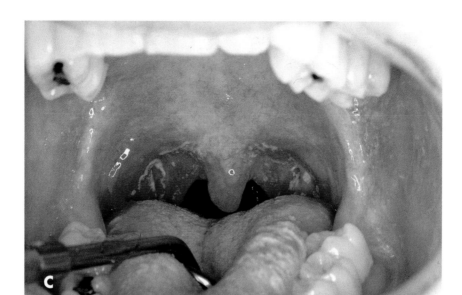

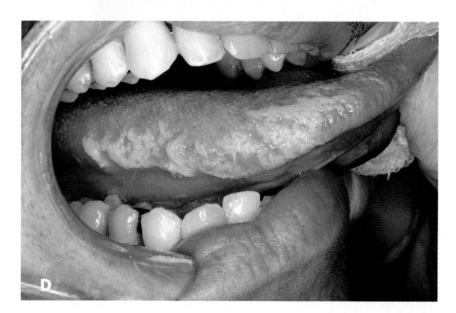

Figure 8.1—cont'd Further examination revealed oropharyngeal candidiasis (**C**) and hairy leukoplakia (**D**). Laboratory tests showed positive HIV serology and skin anergy to four antigens (*Candida,* PPD, mumps, *Trichophyton).*

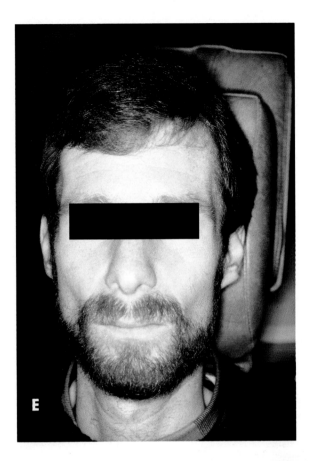

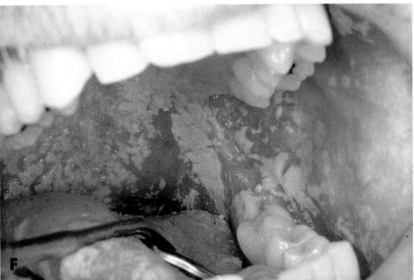

Figure 8.1—cont'd E, Four months later he had lost 30 pounds, developed *Pneumocystis carinii* pneumonia with severe dyspnea, and experienced progressive weakness and malaise. **F,** One month later his oral candidiasis had become florid and refractive to treatment and his T4 lymphocytes fell below $50/mm^3$. He died the following month.

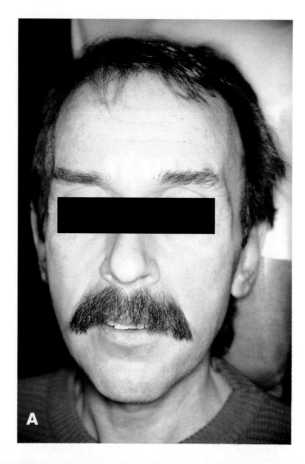

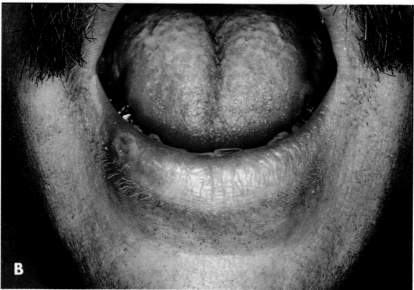

Figure 8.2 A, This 34-year-old AIDS patient complained of dental pain. He has had Kaposi's sarcoma for 1 year, with one bout of *Pneumocystis carinii* pneumonia and some recurrent diarrhea. Examination confirmed herpes labialis **(B).**

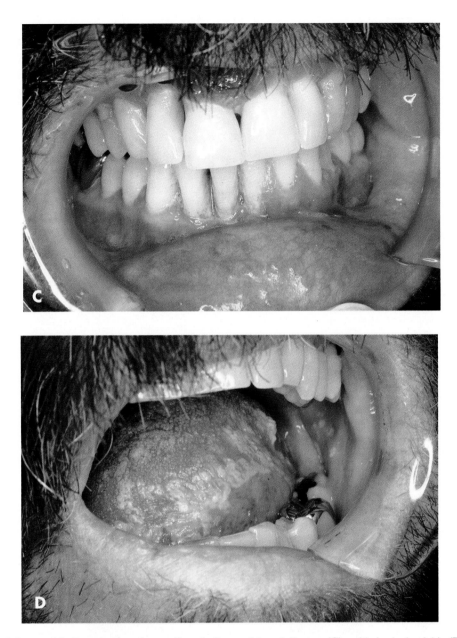

Figure 8.2—cont'd Examination also confirmed advanced dental disease **(C)** and hairy leukoplakia **(D).**

continued

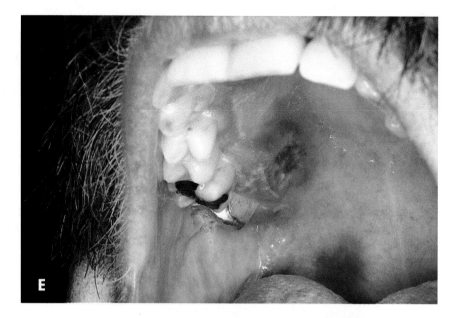

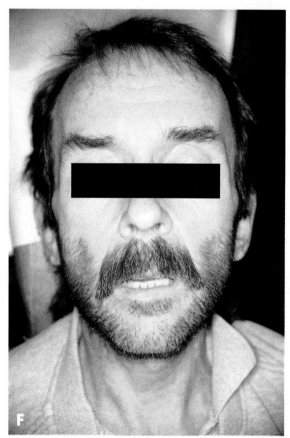

Figure 8.2—cont'd Kaposi's sarcoma of the hard palate was also found, as well as a purpuric lesion (thrombocy-topenia) of the soft palate **(E). F,** He returned 2 weeks later for selected extractions but rapid weight loss, extreme malaise, and weakness precluded any dental work. He died 2 weeks later.

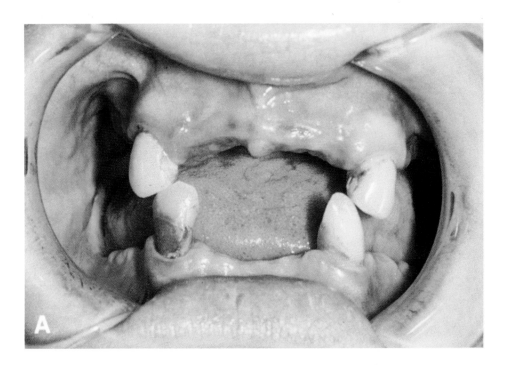

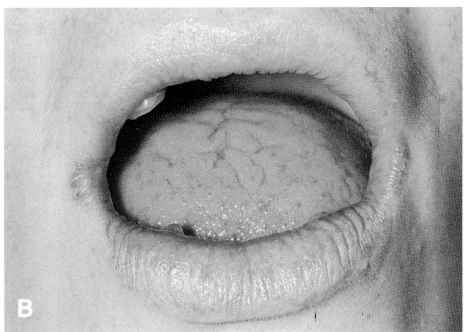

Figure 8.3 This 32-year-old heterosexual female drug addict had been asymptomatic and known to be HIV-positive for 2 years. **A,** She currently is on methadone control and seeking prosthodontic care. She had recently developed symptomatic oral candidiasis. Note the angular cheilitis **(B).**

continued

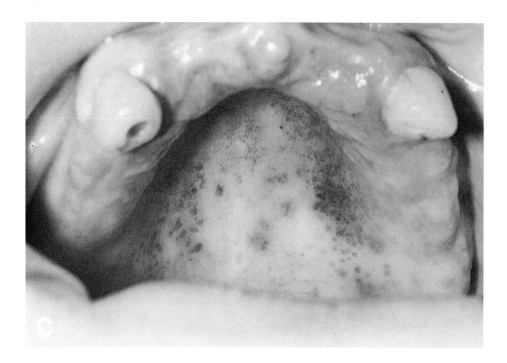

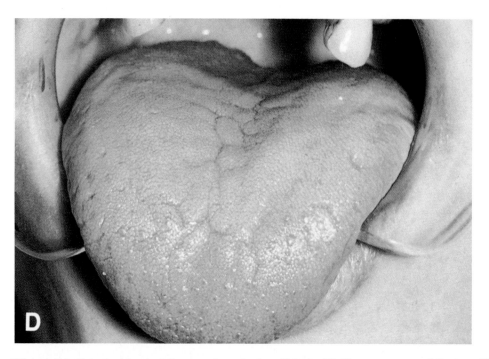

Figure 8.3—cont'd Note the telangiectatic-appearing palatal candidiasis **(C)**. Her tongue was mildly depapillated and sensitive **(D)**. A fungal culture showed heavy growth of *Candida albicans,* which responded to ketoconazole. Her T4 lymphocytes are below 400/mm^3. Of utmost importance, she is in need of counseling. She has an HIV-negative live-in partner who does not use barrier techniques, and she now wants a baby. Obviously, both her partner and baby are at risk of becoming HIV-positive, and her prognosis for survival is poor. She was lost to follow-up.

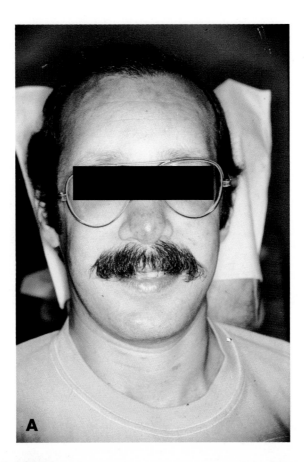

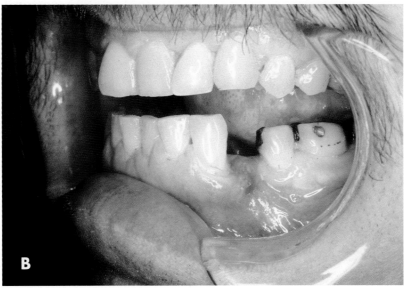

Figure 8.4   A, This 32-year-old street artist presented to the clinic because of a "tooth ache" in his edentulous lower left first bicuspied area. Otherwise he claimed to be in good health and jogged daily. The vascular-appearing lesions and nodules on the skin of his head and neck were characteristic of Kaposi's sarcoma. **B,** Intraoral examination revealed an early Kaposi's sarcoma involving the area of his chief complaint. He was counseled regarding his condition, which was confirmed by positive HIV serology and biopsy. He was referred to the adult immunodeficiency clinic for further evaluation.

continued

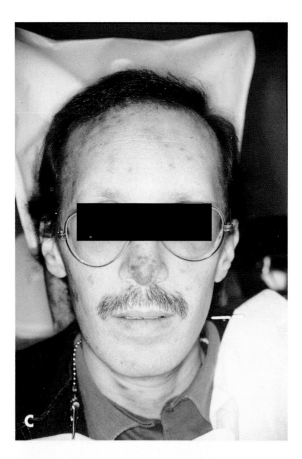

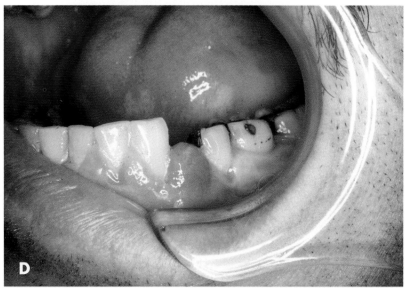

Figure 8.4—cont'd   C, Three months later immunosuppression progressed rapidly, leaving him markedly cachectic and weak. **D,** His intraoral Kaposi's sarcoma progressed and became more bothersome. He died 2 months later.

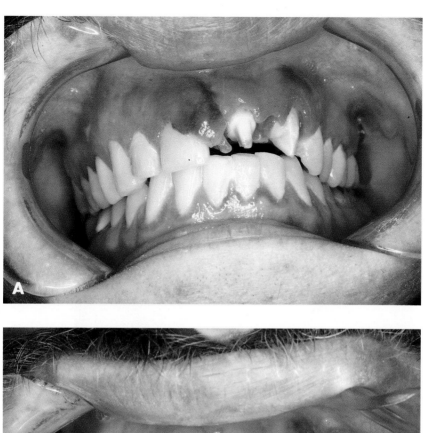

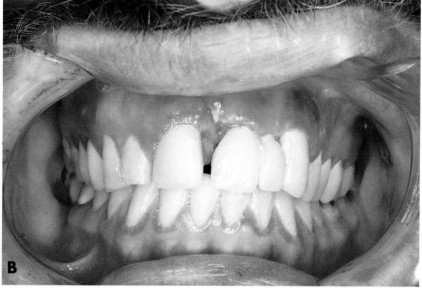

Figure 8.5 This AIDS patient had just lost his anterior bridge. Note the Kaposi's sarcoma of the maxilla, and HIV-associated linear erythema of the mandibular marginal gingiva (**A**). The Kaposi's lesion was excised by CO_2 laser and the bridge recemented (**B**). The patient survived for an additional 6 months.

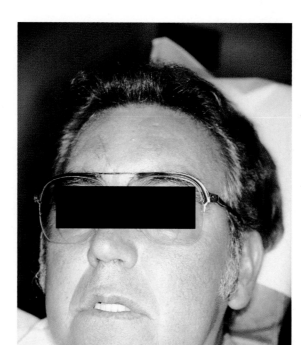

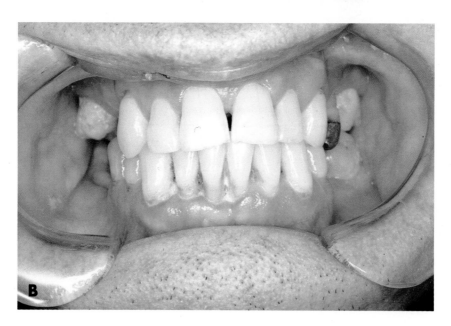

Figure 8.6 A, This 42-year-old bisexual man sought consultation because of a chronically sore mouth for 4 months. He was recently married and had a young daughter, but admitted to previous and some current homosexual activities. **B,** He had peridontosis in spite of a good record of home and office care.

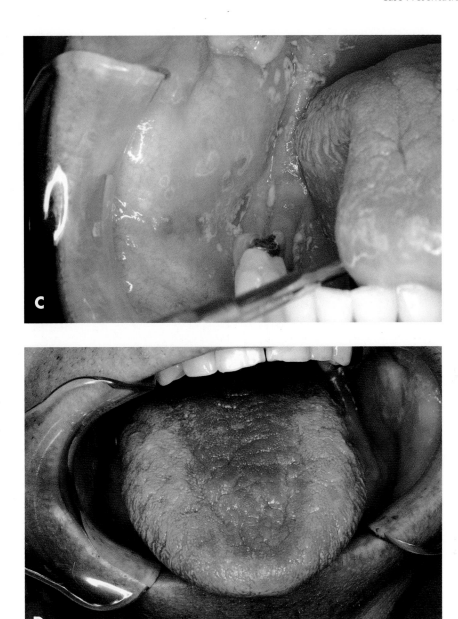

Figure 8.6—cont'd C and **D,** Clinical and laboratory examinations confirmed buccal (pseudomembranous) and tongue (erythematous) lesions of candidiasis. When treated with antifungal medications, both signs and symptoms disappeared.

continued

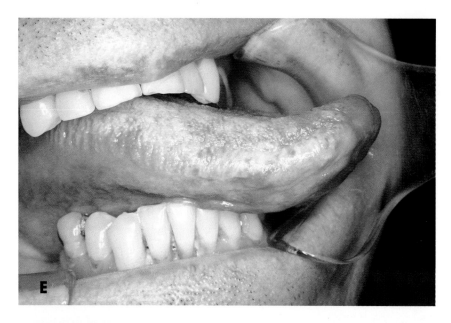

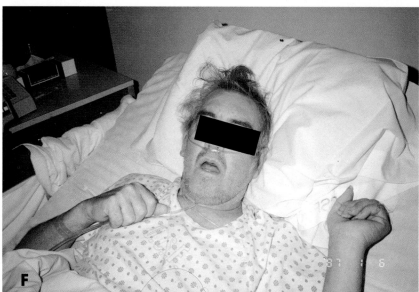

Figure 8.6—cont'd **E,** Hairy leukoplakia was confirmed by biopsy and persisted during antifungal treatment. He was surprised when his serology was HIV-positive. During the following year, his response to antifungal treatment became increasingly refractory. He also developed severe anal candidiasis and intraepithelial carcinoma of the glans penis. He began losing weight rapidly, had bouts of protozoal diarrhea, and developed *Pneumocystis carinii* pneumonia with severe malaise and depression. He and his family asked not to have life support systems, and he died during his second week of hospitalization **(F).**

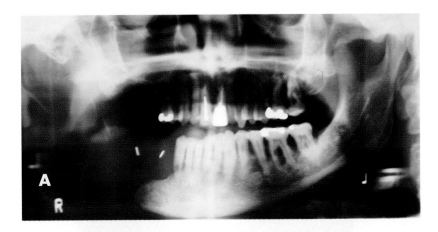

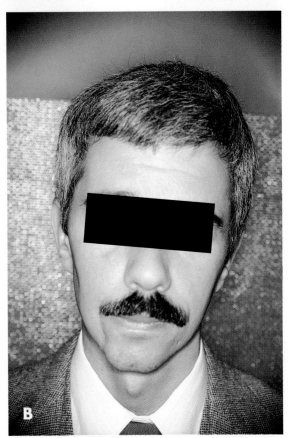

Figure 8.7 A 27-year-old homosexual man developed a squamous carcinoma of the right lateral tongue in 1977. He had a history of hepatitis B, syphilis and gonorrhea, and herpes. He did not use tobacco, alcohol, or "recreational" drugs. Although his tumor responded to radiation therapy, he developed osteonecrosis of his right mandible that did not respond to treatment. **A,** Two years later he had a resection. Note also the periodontal disease. His chronic candidiasis was thought to be due to constant use of antibiotics. **B,** During this period the patient felt well, so 1 year after the resection, he had a muscle graft to improve appearance.

continued

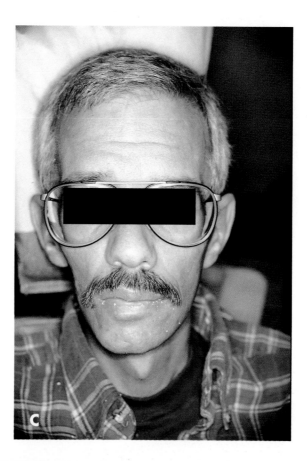

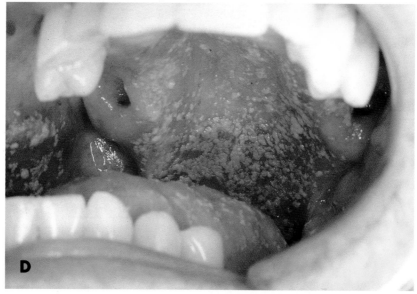

Figure 8.7—cont'd   **C,** and **D,** Four years later, he suddenly developed progressive weight loss, treatment-resistant oral candidiasis, and extreme mobility of teeth and pain. HIV infection was confirmed. The aging process was marked. In a short period of time *Pneumocystis carinii* pneumonia was diagnosed and the patient died. There were no specimens that enabled review of HIV status prior to the progressive wasting syndrome features. Therefore immunosuppression at the time of his early-onset carcinoma can only be speculated.

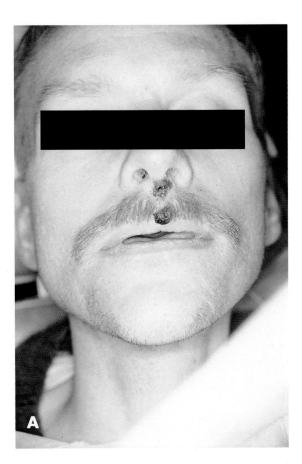

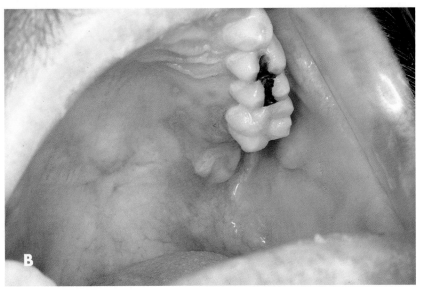

Figure 8.8 This AIDS patient has had chronic genital herpes and was prophylactically on 600 mg acyclovir daily for control. He presented with acute palatal pain. Examination revealed herpetic lesions adjacent to his upper lip and base of nose (**A**) and somewhat typical herpetic ulcerations of his palate (**B**).

continued

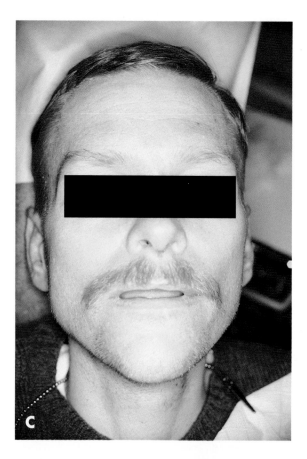

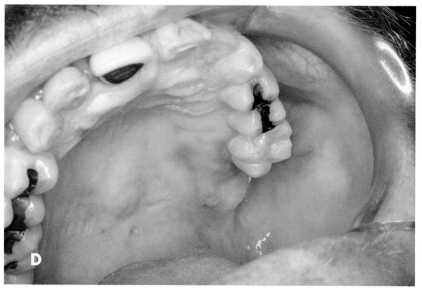

Figure 8.8—cont'd His acyclovir was doubled, and on his return to clinic in 1 week he was asymptomatic and his lesions were essentially cleared (**C** and **D**), at which time the acyclovir was discontinued. It was evident that the herpes strain was becoming thymidine kinase deficient and thus partially resistant to acyclovir.

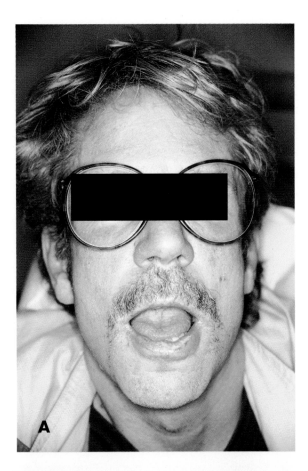

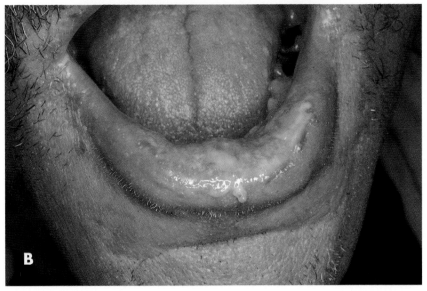

Figure 8.9 This 31-year-old HIV-positive bisexual had been stable for 2 years without any complaints. He was unable to take retroviral drugs because of allergic reactions. His CD4 count was 348. He was referred because of an acute and very painful lip ulceration that had been present for 10 days; it was worsening and precluded adequate dietary intake (**A** and **B**).

continued

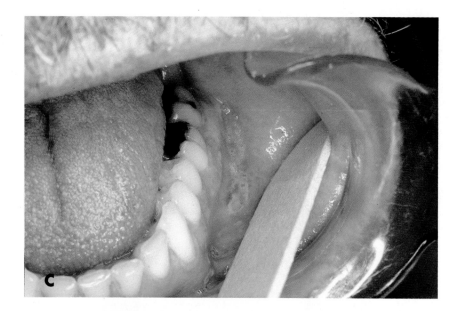

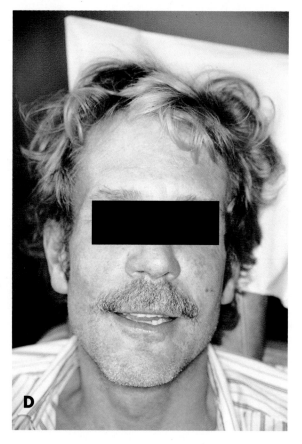

Figure 8.9—cont'd **C,** He also had oral ulcerations. His complaints included excessive weight loss, extreme weakness, and malaise. Based on the history and clinical appearance, the working diagnosis was erythema multiforme. Prednisone (80 mg daily) was instituted. One week later the patient was asymptomatic and healed (**D** to **F**). The prednisone was discontinued; although the patient seemed well, the outbreak forewarned of advancing immunodeficiency.

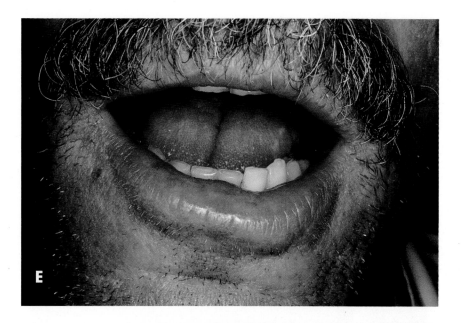

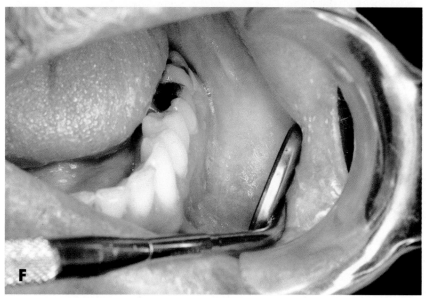

Figure 8.9—cont'd E and **F,** Note the healing after 1 week of prednisone.

continued

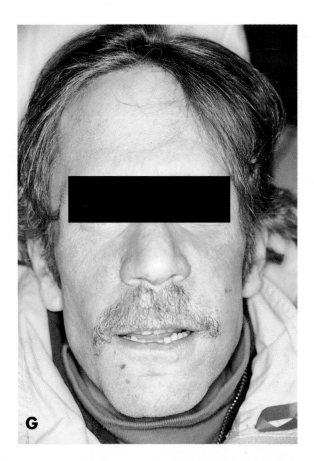

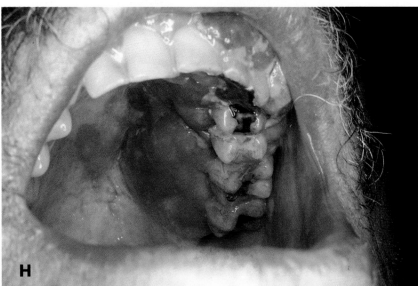

Figure 8.9—cont'd   Fourteen months later other cofactors came into play, his HIV viremia increased, and he progressed into the wasting syndrome along with a flaring hepatitis, oral candidiasis, and oral Kaposi's sarcoma (**G** and **H**). The patient died 2 weeks later.

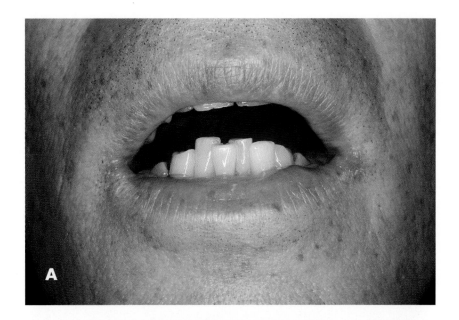

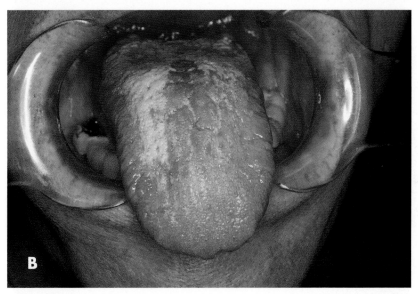

Figure 8.10 A 27-year-old patient with an apparent "negative" medical history was seen because of palatal pain of almost 3 weeks. Clinical findings included angular cheilitis (**A**), an irregularly depapillated tongue (**B**), and diffuse erythematous palatal lesions (**C,** p. 154).

continued

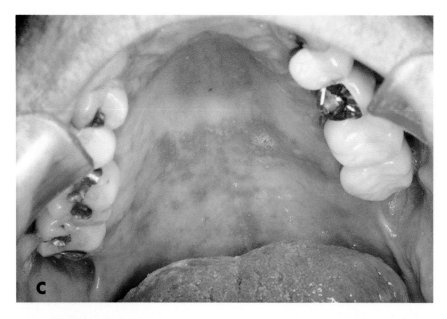

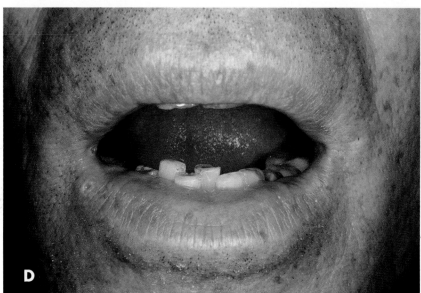

Figure 8.10—cont'd While this suggested several possibilities in the differential diagnosis, candidiasis had the highest priority. He was started on 200 mg ketoconazole once daily with food. **D** to **F,** One week later he returned without any signs and symptoms. Treatment was discontinued, and some signs and symptoms recurred within a month. Immunosuppression was suspicioned, and the patient agreed to HIV testing, which turned out positive. Oral candidiasis was the first sign/symptom of HIV infection that indicated his immune suppression.

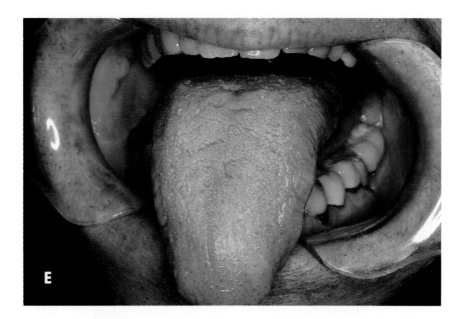

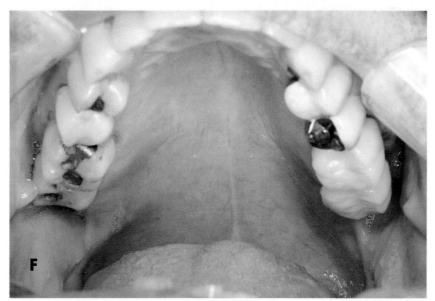

Figure 8.10—cont'd For legend see opposite page.

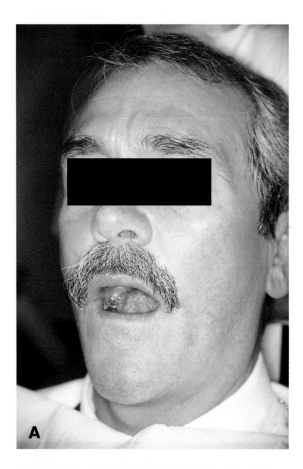

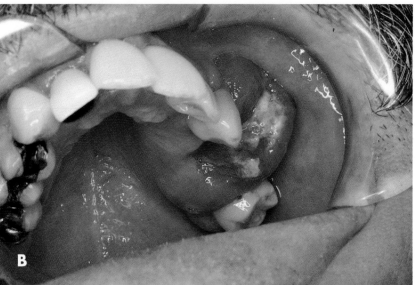

Figure 8.11 A, This 41-year-old homosexual was referred by his dentist because of a 2-week painful swelling of the left maxilla that had not responded to antibiotics and a subsequent extraction. His health history was unremarkable and he had no other complaints or additional information regarding his health. **B,** Examination revealed a large, rubbery-firm mass in the left maxillary molar region. A biopsy specimen was diagnosed as non-Hodgkin's lymphoma (NHL). Because of the large association between NHL and AIDS, he agreed to serologic testing, which resulted in a Western blot confirmation of HIV.

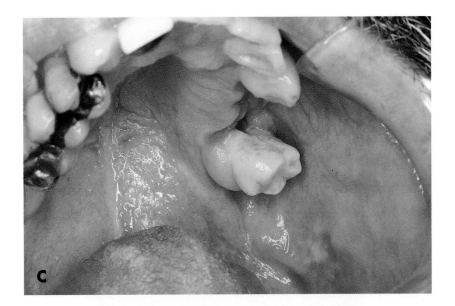

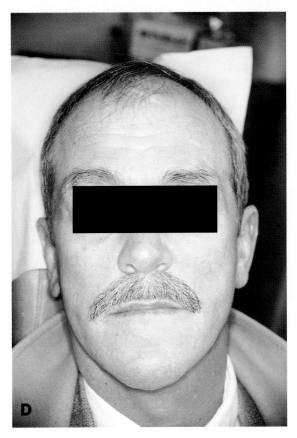

Figure 8.11—cont'd   He was started on an aggressive multidrug 12-week course of chemotherapy. There was a complete response (**C**). The remaining molar was extracted because of advanced bone loss and pain. **D,** Four months later, he progressed into the wasting syndrome (more than 10% unintentional weight loss).

continued

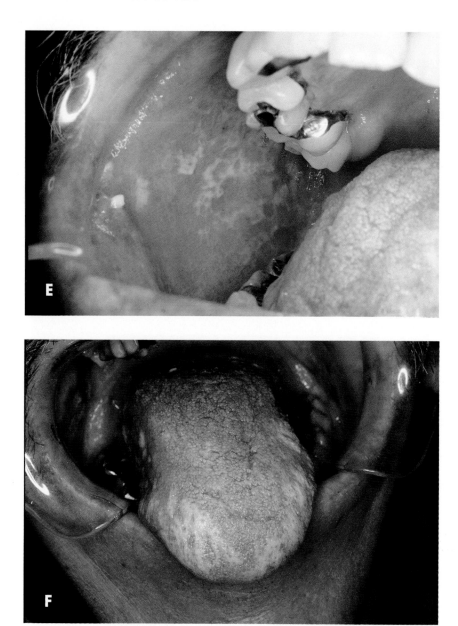

Figure 8.11—cont'd He also developed major aphthae, candidiasis, buccal lichen planus (**E**), and progressive hairy leukoplakia (**F**). He died 2 months later. Only 20% of HIV-associated NHL patients survive 2 years.

INDEX